WUHAN UNION HOSPITAL

The first 84 years

Survival from floods, bombs and enemy confiscation

By
Walford Gillison

Dulverton, England 2015

ISBN-13: 978-1508565680

ISBN-10: 1508565686

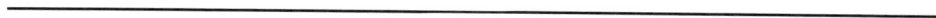

DEDICATION

Professor Ye Huai Ying (Lucy Ye)
(28-09-1920 to 05-06-2014)

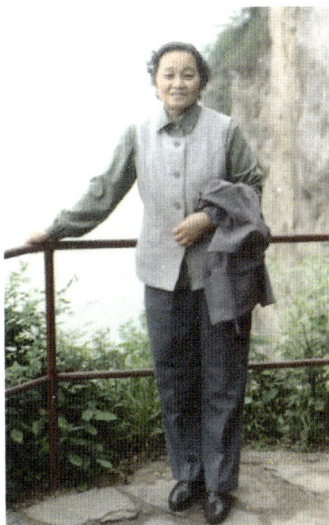

She was born in Wuhan in September 28th, 1920 in a medical family. Her father Dr Ye Kecheng worked in Hankou Renji Hospital (later merged with Union Hospital) for over 40 years. She was deeply influenced by her father when she was young. As described in Chapter 6 her father and Surgeon YK Liu literally saved the Union Hospital from takeover and probable demolition during the years from 1942 to 1944 when Wuhan was under Japanese occupation.

Lucy Ye went to medical school in 1938 at the age of 18 and graduated from West China Medical School of Sichuan University as a medical doctor (M.D.) in 1946. In 1946, Lucy Ye at the age of 26 became an Obstetrics and Gynaecology physician in Wuhan Union Hospital, where she was the first Chinese doctor in that Department. She worked in Wuhan Union Hospital for over 60 years, and carried on even while she was diagnosed and successfully treated for endometrial cancer in 2008.

She married to Professor Gao Yu who was a very famous Cardiovascular physician in China in 1956 and both of them devoted their lifetime services to Wuhan Union Hospital. In 1985, she resigned from her substantive post, but continued to visit her old wards and participate in research. She didn't fully retire until 2009. She saw outpatients regularly until 2008.

On March 25th, 2012 Prof. Ye Huai Ying, at the age of 91, decided to donate her house and property to her own charity "THE GAO YU, YE HUAI YING AND GAO JINGXING EDUCATION FUND". This charity was designed to support poverty-stricken students while attending the Department of Gynaecology and Obstetrics as well as the Cardiovascular Institute. According to her wish, after her death her house was to be sold, the proceeds to go to a bursary in order to support 8 to 10 students from humble backgrounds each with a grant of 6,000 Yuan per year.

As a doctor for over 60 years, Prof. Ye always treated her patients as if they were relatives or personal friends. At one time she was an honorary director of Hubei Genetic Medical Center and had gained many honours from the Ministries of Education and Health. Moreover, she trained the first group of graduate students in Gynaecology and Obstetrics in China, at least five of them are now working in various institutes in the United States of America.

During her life she was a warm-hearted friend to people of all ages, all sections of society and to visitors of all nationalities who came to visit the hospital over many years.

She died at the age of 93, loved by many and will be sorely missed.

ACKNOWLEDGEMENTS

I wish to thank several members of the staff of the Wuhan Union Hospital not only for their generosity to my family, but for stimulating the idea of a written record of the early days before the institution became State controlled in 1950 after 84 years of struggle for survival by private donations and private enterprise.

I thank Wuhan graduate Dr Dunsong Yang, a senior scientist in the Florida Institute for Reproductive Medicine and Prof Ye's stepdaughter Peggy Udel for details and accuracy of the Dedication.

I am grateful to President and senior surgeon Wang Guobin for the hospitality given to me and my family on three occasions since 2001. Therefore it is with pleasure that I shall present him with all my material for his scholars to translate my humble offering into Chinese.

I and my family are very aware of the complete change in the atmosphere from 65 years ago when my parents and other foreign members of the staff had to leave Wuhan in haste in 1950. At that time they were forced to leave their medical and nursing colleagues abruptly with whom lifelong friendships had been made. They were not sorry to leave the imposed political new members of staff who made life difficult by actively discouraging social contacts and friendships with their Chinese colleagues.

The atmosphere now is completely different since the beginning of the 21st century. Besides President Guobin Wang, I can regard people like Hongbo Wang (Associate Director of International affairs) Jianjun Wang (Head of Thoracic Surgery) Xiaogang Shu Associate Professor of Gastrointestinal Surgery and Dr Feng Gao from the

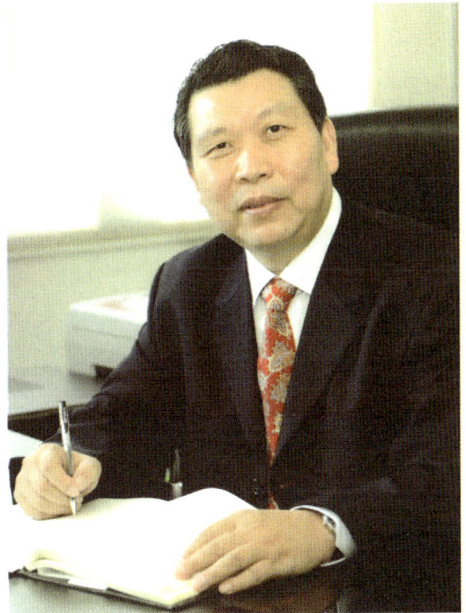

President Wang Guobin

v

Department of Administration as personal friends. I am grateful for the excellent photographs taken by our family friend Hao Zhou who is at present Associate Professor in the Department of Haematology. His illustrations are shown on the back cover.

I am obliged to Audrey Salters who took the material from her mother's letters to tell the story of the vicious Sino-Japanese war taking place in North China at the same time as my father had to work in the Union Hospital under scrutiny of the Japanese. Her book "Bound with Love" was another stimulus to me to record some of the events along the Yangtse River during the Second Sino-Japanese War.

I am obliged to Joanne Ichimura, Archivist Archives & Special Collections at the Library at the School of Oriental and African Studies (SOAS) and her staff in Russell Square in London. There is now a useful collection of documents and correspondence between several Missionary Societies and their staff working in other countries besides China.

Dr Jocelyn Chatterton from London's School of Oriental and African studies has been of tremendous help in filling in the events between my leaving Hankou on August 13th 1942 until my father's return in 1947.

I am obliged to Ceri Keene who designed and created figures 9 and 11 in the main story as well as the modified map showing the protagonists during the Second Sino-Japanese War. (Figure 4, second appendix).

I am grateful to Jane Erith too for her meticulous approach to proof reading and also my sister Fran Clemmow for reading and advice of earlier drafts. Claire Savill is not only an artist but has applied her experience in the science of printing. Claire put the text and illustrations together and made the major negotiations with the publisher.

Last but by no means least I want to give thanks to my wife Sue who over the last 46 years has been a source of strength, common sense and encouragement for this book in the same manner that she has for my career as a surgeon. I am convinced without her this book would never have been written.

Walford Gillison. 2015.

FOREWORD

WUHAN UNION HOSPITAL:
The first 84 years.

First of all there is a conflict in terminology which can be explained by the drastic changes in history as a result of a complete change in the ideology of the nation of China. Hankow is now spelt Hankou, but until 1950 it was known as the "Hankow Union Hospital". However after the complete ideological change in the government of all China except Taiwan, the State took the Hospital over and expanded it to become a fine Teaching Hospital as well as a medical centre providing all-round care to the City of Wuhan and the surrounding province of Hubei. Now it is known as the "Wuhan Union Hospital".

I was born in the Hankou Union Hospital in Central China in 1935. In 2016 the Hospital will be celebrating its 150th anniversary. This factor alone is a good reason for getting some historical record written down before all memories and records are lost. To assist the occasional reader I have shown many of the dates clearly throughout the text for speed and convenience.

I apologise for the surgical bias in this account. Perhaps it is because until 1950 my father was a member of the surgical staff in that hospital and I happened to follow in his footsteps in surgery many years later in the United Kingdom. There is an imbalance of the events which are biased towards the Gillison family which could not be helped. So much historical material came from my father, Keith Gillison, which can be found in his autobiography "The Cross and the Dragon"[1]. Some further details came from the recent discovery of diaries written from 1928 to 1945 by my mother (Kathleen Gillison). I am much indebted to my sister Fran who spent many years cataloguing a surprising cache of family letters related to our grandparents who spent the major part of their lives as medical missionaries working in and around the Wuhan Union Hospital in China. Fran has summarised the cache into a very readable book mentioned below.[2]

It is sad that many of the pioneers intimately associated with the Union Hospital are deceased. There are so many unanswered questions that I would have liked to have asked, but has been unable to do so.

I wish to declare my gratitude for much of the material gained from the PhD thesis by Dr Jocelyn Chatterton submitted to the School of Oriental and African Studies (SOAS) in London[3]. The quantity and depth of detail in her work is an example to any researcher on a complex historical study. I shall always be in her debt. That material is available to anyone applying for access to the SOAS website.

Finally as with all revolutions, destruction of records has taken place since the advent of the new ideology introduced by Chairman Mao and the new government of modern China in 1950. This has made research on the earlier history of the hospital more difficult.

I trust the reader will find this record of some interest as the changes in Union Hospital have been reflected in the changes in the whole of China. There is absolutely no doubt that the staff of the Union Hospital can be proud of the huge advances since the Government of China took over the running of the hospital in 1950. I hope, on looking back at the history, the same staff today can be equally proud of the dedication, sacrifices and determination for the survival of the same hospital that had taken place over the previous 84 years.

Walford Gillison 2015

1. Keith Gillison: "The Cross and the Dragon, a medical family in China" Published and printed by Hawthornes of Nottingham 1988

2. Clemmow Frances: "Days of sorrow, Times of Joy"
The story of a Victorian family's love affair with China
Matador 2012

3. Jocelyn Chatterton "Protestant Medical Missionary Experience during the War in China 1937–1945: The Case of Hubei Province" PhD Thesis
School of Oriental and African Studies, University of London 2010

TERMINOLOGY

The Wade-Giles system of romanising the modern Chinese written language was originally devised to simplify Chinese-language characters for Westerners. It was first initiated by Sir Thomas Francis Wade and then modified by professor Herbert Allen Giles at the University of Cambridge in his *Chinese-English Dictionary* of 1912. With Giles's syllabic changes, Wade-Giles became the preferred Chinese transliteration system among both academics and non-specialists in the English-speaking world and was interpreted into Danish, Finnish, German, Italian, Norwegian, Spanish, Swedish, and Turkish. The Chinese themselves experimented with several systems to transcribe local expressions for non-Chinese publications but in mainland China these were all replaced officially in 1979 by the clearer **Pinyin** romanisation system. The Wade-Giles system continued to be used in Taiwan, although a modified system somewhat between Pinyin and Wade-Giles has been in limited use since about 2000.

From the point of view of the early history of the Wuhan Union Hospital, the Pinyin terms will be used but the Wade-Giles spelling will be put in parentheses on the first occasion, to be followed only by the modern Pinyin spellings for the rest of the story. Below is the list of people or places that are mentioned in the book.

Pinyin	Wade-Giles
Beijing	Peking
Chongqing	Chunking
Guangzhou	Canton
Hangzhou	Hangchow
Hankou	Hankow
Jiang Jieshi	Chiang Kai Shek
Jinan	Tsinan
Jiujiang	Kiukiang
Lushan	Kuling
Manzhouguo	Manchukuo*
Mao Zedong	Mao Tse Tung
Nanjing	Nanking
Pudong	Pootung
Xiaogan	Hsiao Gan
Tianjin	Tientsin
Yangzhou	Yangchow
Yichang	Ichang
Zhenjiang	Chinkiang

* In the English speaking world this region was known as Manchuria, for simplicity this name out of the three, is used in the text describing the Second Sino-Japanese War.

CONTENTS

WUHAN UNION HOSPITAL. The First 84 Years.

ILLUSTRATIONS

CHAPTER 1

WUHAN UNION HOSPITAL: 1866 to 1950

EARLY IMPERIALIST TIMES

1866 – 1882

The principal move to form a district General Hospital came from a British Protestant preacher called Griffith John (figure 1). He was an eloquent public speaker, preacher and tireless worker. He believed that he should spend his entire working life in Central China to introduce Christianity to the local people of China and generate an understanding of a different culture to the nineteenth-century people of China. He stayed in Shanghai until 1860, unable to move inland until that year when the Tianjin (Tientsin) Treaty was signed (Appendix 1; Summary of the Opium Wars and Christian missionary societies) which allowed him to move, live and work where he believed that God required him to be; in other words in Central China.

He arrived to start his life's work in Hankou which was then and still is part of the bigger metropolis of Wuhan (figure 2). He left Shanghai on June 9th and was pleased to step off the ship called the "Hellespont" on the dry land of Hankou on June 21st 1861[1]. After exploring the region for several weeks he became convinced it was the place to spend his whole working life. Therefore he went back to Shanghai, and collected his wife and two very tender aged sons in order to set up his first home in China that September.

Figure 1

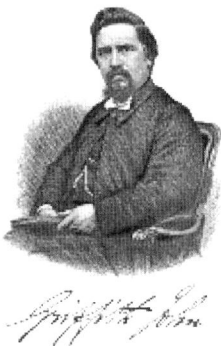

Griffith John 1831 – 1912

From: Griffith John: The Story of Fifty Years in China
p.272
London The Religious Tract Society:
Bouverie St, & 65 St. Paul's Churchyard, EC
(Popular revised edition 1908)

Though he believed his life task was to preach Christianity in Central China, he had always believed since his arrival in 1861 there was a strong need to have:

1. A church building for preaching and worship
2. A school or an educational centre for young and old
3. A proper hospital rather than a small dispensary and first aid centre[2] . (After prompting by local residents and riverside personnel).

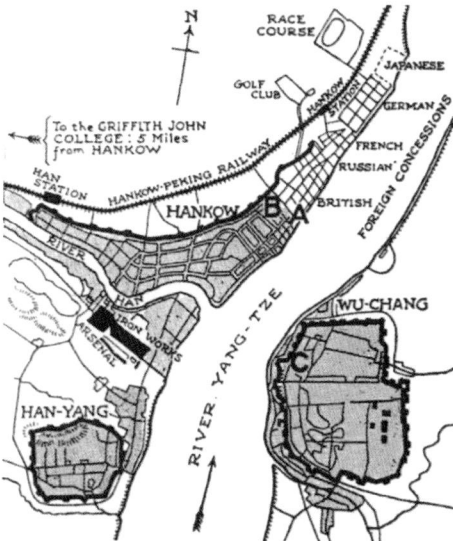

Figure 2.

Foreign concessions on the Yangtse River in 1904
From: Griffith John: The Story of Fifty Years in China p272 London (The original Wade-Giles spelling is maintained)

Wuhan has been understandably divided into three parts because of the joining of the Han River almost at right angles to the great Yangtse River shown in figure 2.

1. Hankou
2. Wuchang
3. Hanyang

Hankou became the main centre for trade and international relations. Wuchang was the seat of local government and Hanyang became famous for industrial development after the Peking government exploited an iron ore foundry and other industrial enterprises.

Before the building of the Three Gorges Dam was completed in 2014, the River Yangtse had been at times a mile in width in spring and early summer due to the melting of the snows in the Himalayas far away to the west. It is because of its width and navigability that foreign concessions, functioning like minor embassies of the British, Russian, French, German and Japanese legations, were established after the Tianjin treaty of 1856 described in the first Appendix.

At last in 1866 Griffith John was able to enlist the willing help of Dr Arthur G Reid, physician to the British Concession, to form the nucleus of a medical centre in Hankou. This physician had not only taken the trouble to learn Chinese but gave his services free of charge two days a week for several years. The early centre began as a simple clinic but in 1873 Dr Reid organised two wards each containing 25 male and 25 female beds[3]. Male and female patients had to be doctored and nursed separately in those days. Added to that, he enlisted the help of two dedicated servants whom he had already trained in basic nursing skills. This was 43 years before the founding of the Nursing Association of China.

In 1870 Dr Shearer arrived and acted as medical officer for two and a half years. This released Dr Reid to return to his medical duties at the British Concession. However Dr Shearer, for reasons unexplained, left Hankou and went into private medical practice in Jiujiang (Kiukiang). Dr Reid returned to continue the same service two days a week for the next five years. He was also responsible for the "erection of a much larger and more suitable hospital"[2]. In 1874 funds in the order of £1350.00, a huge amount of money those days, from both Chinese and foreign Church sources from all over the world were collected to build larger premises.

Sadly the health of Griffith John's first wife Margaret (figure 3) badly deteriorated due to heart failure so Dr John took her back to the United States for medical assessment and treatment on their way to the United Kingdom. At the end of their leave in 1873 Margaret was still determined to return with her husband back to China no matter the state of her health. As it happened she died on board the ship SS Hector entering Singapore harbour on the journey back to Hankou[4] on the 24th March 1873.

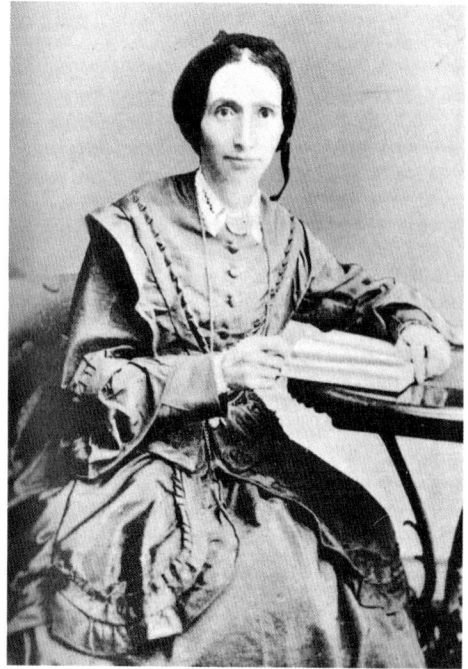

Figure 3

Portrait of Margaret John

Thompson R. Wardlaw
Griffith John: The story of 50 years in
China p300
London The Religious Tract Society:
Bouverie St &
65 St. Paul's Churchyard EC
(Popular revised edition 1908)

In 1874 it was agreed that a larger building was needed for the increased medical work, so larger premises were found. As a tribute to her memory Griffith John collected sufficient money to expand the women's ward completing a dedicated building to be called "The Margaret John Women's Hospital". By 1891 this female wing, added to the men's ward, increased the capacity of this embryonic hospital from 50 to 60 beds.

During the years of 1875 to 1879 a new doctor, Kenneth McKenzie, was appointed who worked full-time in Hankou for four years[5]. He helped to increase the inpatient and outpatient work on the site so that in 1875 1800 new outpatient consultations were recorded in which 33 inpatients had operations including 6 foreign sailors. Out of interest two patients had cataract operations.

The total medical care in Hankou City at that time comprised:

- Five General Hospitals
- Two women's hospitals, including the developing Margaret John wing
- One leprosy asylum

4

From 1879 to 1883 William George Mawbey (who excised a shoulder joint for severe tuberculosis; a very remarkable operation in those days) arrived and replaced Dr McKenzie. Dr Wang Kien Tang who had been trained by Drs McKenzie, Reid and Shearer joined the medical team in a part-time capacity. Soon after, Dr Tang opened his own private hospital nearby but provided part time help. In other emergency situations Dr Begg from Wuchang worked part-time until the expected arrival of Dr Tom Gillison in 1883.

1882 – 1894

While grateful for the help of the above-mentioned doctors, Griffith John was at last able to find someone to provide a more permanent medical commitment. Tom Gillison (figure 4) arrived in Shanghai at the end of 1882 and he visited an Edinburgh medical contemporary in Jiujiang before arriving in Hankou. He steadfastly set himself to learn Chinese for six months before full-time clinical duties. Needless to say he had to pitch in to the medical work when both his colleagues were away due to sickness or leave. His actual contract started on May 1st 1883.

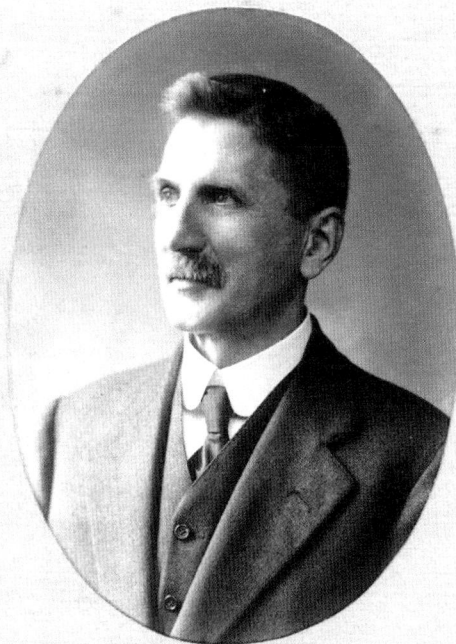

Figure 4

Tom Gillison as a young man.

(Gillison family photographs.)

In 1883 Dr Mawbey decided to return to the UK following the sudden unknown cause of death of his wife in Hankou, leaving Tom Gillison on his own.

By 1887 over 2000 outpatients were seen and the two establishments of the combined Men's wing and Margaret John wing fully utilised those precious 50 inpatient beds, with ten mattresses on the floors which could be used for emergencies.

In 1890 Dr AM Mackay, mainly based in Wuchang, came to work part-time at the Union Hospital alongside Tom Gillison, and later Dr Percy Lonsdale McAll joined them. The inpatient work had increased so much that they were forced to abandon routine home visits because it took precious time away from the hospital. This change was regretted because in those days so many patients preferred to be seen in their own homes rather than possibly a forbidding foreign-looking establishment.

1891 marked the year of the official founding of the Margaret John Memorial Hospital for women, when the building of the new premises had begun. However it took another eight years (1899) before the building was complete and formal care of the patients took place.

Admissions due to opium addiction were a very dominant cause of pressure on the hospital beds for many subsequent years. A major crisis had arisen through the prolific growing of opium poppies for many miles around in Hubei, causing many more inpatient and outpatient consultations as a result. One day, when a foreign staff member was talking to a local farmer who linked all foreigners with commercial opium production, this man understandably said: "You foreigners have profited by the opium hitherto, so we are determined to cut you out of it and obtain the benefit from it ourselves"[6]. (See the Opium Wars and the relation to China missionaries in the first Appendix).

On a happier note, on September 7th 1893 Dr Tom Gillison married Dr Elizabeth May (Bessie) Harris (Figure 5) at the British Consulate. He had met her the previous year on leave in the UK. She was one of the early graduates from the women's Royal Free Hospital in London and since her schooldays had been determined to come out to China and work as a medical missionary. Dr Mackay acted as best man to Tom Gillison at the ceremony and he also covered Tom's medical duties in Hankou for the short time while the wedding couple spent their honeymoon in Wuchang.

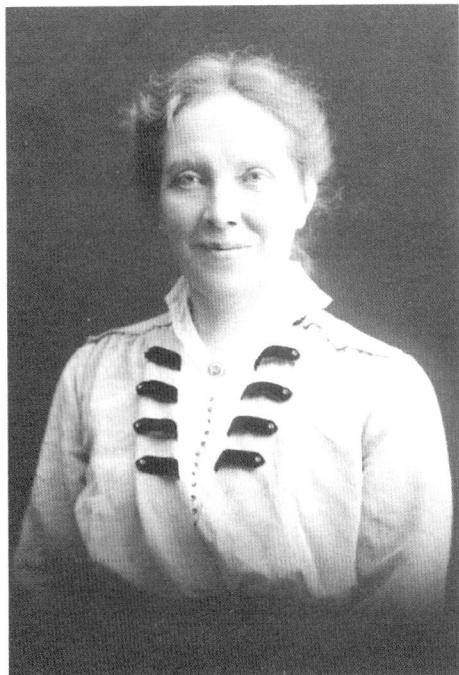

Figure 5

**Elizabeth (Bessie) May Gillison née Harris.
(1869 – 1936)**
(Gillison family archives.)

In 1894 both Tom and Bessie Gillison contracted typhoid fever, a risk so many foreigners took, so they were forced to take sick leave in Japan for a few months before coming back to work. On return to Hankou Bessie Gillison started work in the new Margaret Memorial Hospital until the birth of her first child Edwin Walford in 1894.

1895 – 1901

1895 was a year during which there was tremendous heat in June and July, coinciding with Tom and Bessie Gillison becoming ill, this time with dysentery. Hankou in mid-summer for foreigners was a dangerous time as regards infectious diseases. This was sufficiently serious for them to arrange sick leave in England. Tom recovered surprisingly quickly and was back to work in a few months.

In the meantime help in the Women's Hospital came from newly appointed Dr AL Cousins and senior Nurse Wylie. Male patients continued to be treated in a separate building called the "Men's Hospital". By the end of 1895, 2270 outpatients had been seen and 93 inpatients treated in both hospital wings, which included 36 chloroform anaesthetics[7]. Chloroform was found to be more useful in hot climates because the alternative inhalant ether, an agent among anaesthetists with a safer reputation, had a more volatile vapour and was found to be more difficult to induce and maintain anaesthesia in the summer heat [8].

In 1896 Dr Ernest Turner arrived in Hankou to join Tom Gillison but within a few weeks both he and Tom contracted Typhus. Dr Turner died but Tom Gillison recovered. The toll on new arrivals from infection in those pre-antibiotic days was often severe. To make matters worse Dr Mackay died from cholera when he returned to Wuchang. While these pioneers knew the dangers in living in Central China, it is a tribute to their courage as well as their dedication that so many risked their lives to these infectious diseases. They all shared the unshakable determination that God wanted them to live and work in China.

The Boxer Rebellion started in 1899 and continued into 1900 and 1901. News of the rebellion reached Wuhan and caused considerable anxiety. Owing to violence elsewhere in China[9] there were reported deaths of at least 250 foreigners and probably several thousand Chinese Christians. Therefore in June 1900, when Tom and Bessie's second son Keith was born, Tom sent Bessie and her children to Japan until the social and political upheaval settled down[10]. In fact life returned to normal in just a few weeks, so the family and several other foreign refugees were able to return to their work and domestic duties in Hankou as before.

1902 – 1912

1902 was the year that the Union Hospital Medical School[11] was founded. It was to be a medical school to train young Chinese doctors in modern medicine combined with strong ethical principles. This dream was to become true for Doctors Gillison and McAll (figure 6). Their aim was that medical students from China could graduate and practise medicine not only in Wuhan but all over China. The intake was small, at first only 9 students,

8

but it was a start and it was to become the nucleus of a great centre of medical education. Of these nine medical students only one could afford the full tuition fees. The others were trusted to pay and did pay for their studies after graduation

Figure 6

**Dr. Percy Lonsdale McAll
(1870-1937)**
Courtesy of his granddaughter
Elizabeth Lester

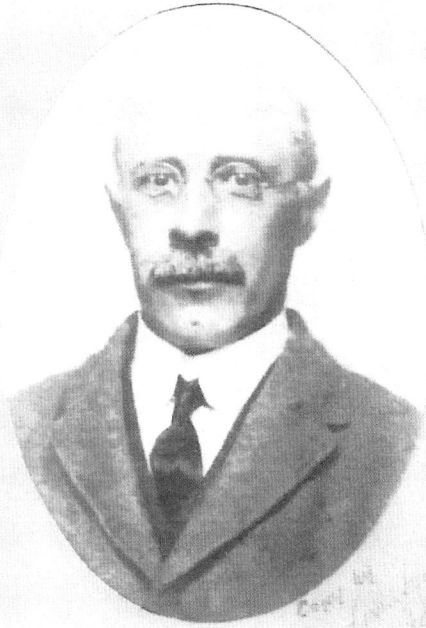

A syllabus was set up emphasising the following points:

- Four years of systematic teaching followed by two years working in the hospital wards
- The teaching was to be in the Chinese language
- Admission of students offered to Christians and also young people of good moral character
- To train more Christian Chinese medical missionaries but an "open door" to deserving non-Christian students was offered as well
- The ultimate purpose was one day to link with other doctors in Wuhan to make a larger Medical School

In 1907 Hilda Margaret Byles arrived in Hankou. She was another dedicated missionary doctor sent out by the London Missionary Society, who wanted specifically to contribute to the medical work in the Margaret

John Memorial Hospital. She believed God wanted her to specialise in the obstetric services.

Figure 7

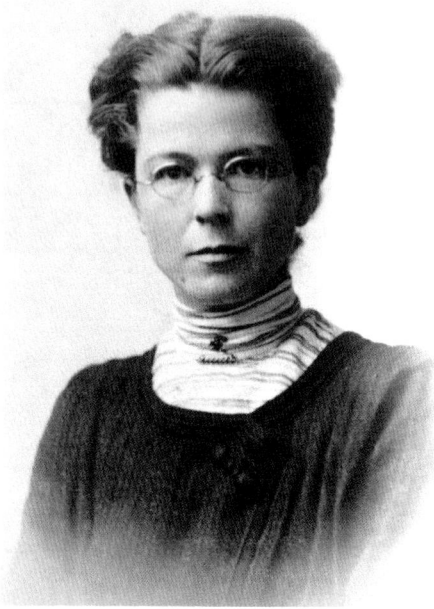

Hilda Margaret Byles, M.B., B.S. London. (1871 – 1931)
(Courtesy of School of Oriental and African Studies (SOAS) in London).

Like Bessie Gillison, Hilda Byles was a graduate of the Royal Free Hospital in London which was the only medical school in England to enable women to graduate as doctors in those days. She always regarded herself as a friend of the Chinese people; she supported the republican aspirations in China and was a tireless worker in the Margaret John Hospital. As the majority of Chinese women in those days preferred to have their babies at home, Hilda Byles introduced a programme specifically to teach nurses safe obstetric procedures for home confinements. She later co-founded the Domiciliary Obstetric Association of China.

Besides her passion for high quality obstetrics, she was also known as a defender of helpless young women. Many young girls orphaned by disease or disaster could easily be forced into a life of prostitution. Kathleen Gillison, in one of her later diaries[12], described how a few of them managed to escape the brothel keepers but they were only safe in the Union Hospital for a limited time before pressure through local courts could be applied to retrieve them. It was not uncommon for these brothel keepers to camp on the doorstep of the Margaret John Hospital wing and demand the return of these pathetic sources of revenue. Providentially Dr Byles had made a valuable contact with a hostel in Shanghai to which these destitute girls and young women could escape. Similar hostels in other parts of China were established and these hostels where such girls could make lives of their own were called "Doors of Hope".

In 1911 The Union Hospital's first matron (Miss Hope Bell) who had trained at the London Hospital (now the Royal London Hospital) was appointed. She made considerable contributions to the Nursing Association of China which was founded in 1912 and she started the official training of men into the Nursing Profession in Central China. She was President of the Nursing Association of China in 1914 and 1915 and later Secretary of the Association in 1926 to 1928. She retired and returned to the UK in 1931 and lived until 1968.

Figure 8

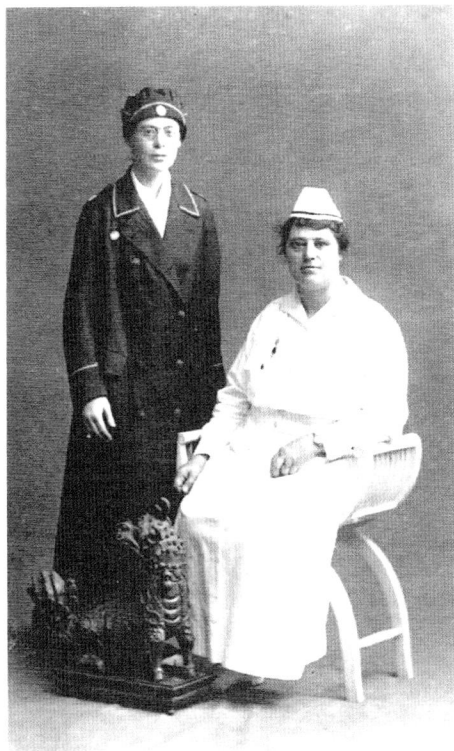

Miss Hope Bell first matron of the Union hospital is standing next to the seated Cora Simpson, one of the founding members of the Nursing Association of China
(Courtesy of SOAS in London)

1911-12 heralded the beginning of the revolution against the Manchu Imperial dynasty and the foundation of the Republic of China. The official date was October 10th colloquially known as the "Double Tenth". It started with the burning of Law courts and police stations in Wuchang along with the slaughtering of many Manchu officials. The same rebellion spread to Hankou and Hanyang. The Red Cross quickly bought in medical supplies and food and set up several temporary casualty stations.

Tom Gillison was rightly proud of many of the Union Hospital students who either helped working in the hospital or in the emergency Red Cross centres in the city centre. He estimated at least 200 casualties were admitted to the Union Hospital during those three days of bitter fighting. The staff was forced to convert the church premises into a triage centre before sending the wounded to the operating theatre, to those 60 precious beds, the mortuary or elsewhere.

Below is the summary of Tom Gillison's main account[13] written to his son Walford, after whom I was later named, when he was at school in Scotland. Tom Gillison's map is modified and shown here in figure 9.

"Some of the students had left but many stayed on to help the Red Cross in the city and help in the Hospital. One was mindful that there were several (Chinese) Imperial ships moored a few miles down the Yangtse River.

The Imperial troops raided Railway station A and captured it after a big battle and next went on to Station B which they captured. The battle went on for three and a half days before they captured "Boundary Road" (possibly Sin Sen Road) years later on November 1st.

Hundreds were killed and over a thousand injured. There were over two hundred of the injured admitted into the 60 bedded Union Hospital on the first day. The Hospital Church acted as a recovery ward to help the crush of admissions. As bullets and mortars were occasionally fired down the Boundary Road, sesame seed bags were made into a barrier to allow civilians to cross the road from their homes to the hospital.

Whether as a result of the shelling or by deliberate intent, the city of Hankow was set on fire which then contained about 40,000 inhabitants whereas normally there would be 500,000. Of great concern to everyone was the fear that there were 150 patients in the Wesleyan Hospital trapped in the centre of the conflagration.

At first the imperial troops were victorious; they shot any looters of empty property and even killed any adult male not displaying a pig-tail or queue denoting support for the Emperor".

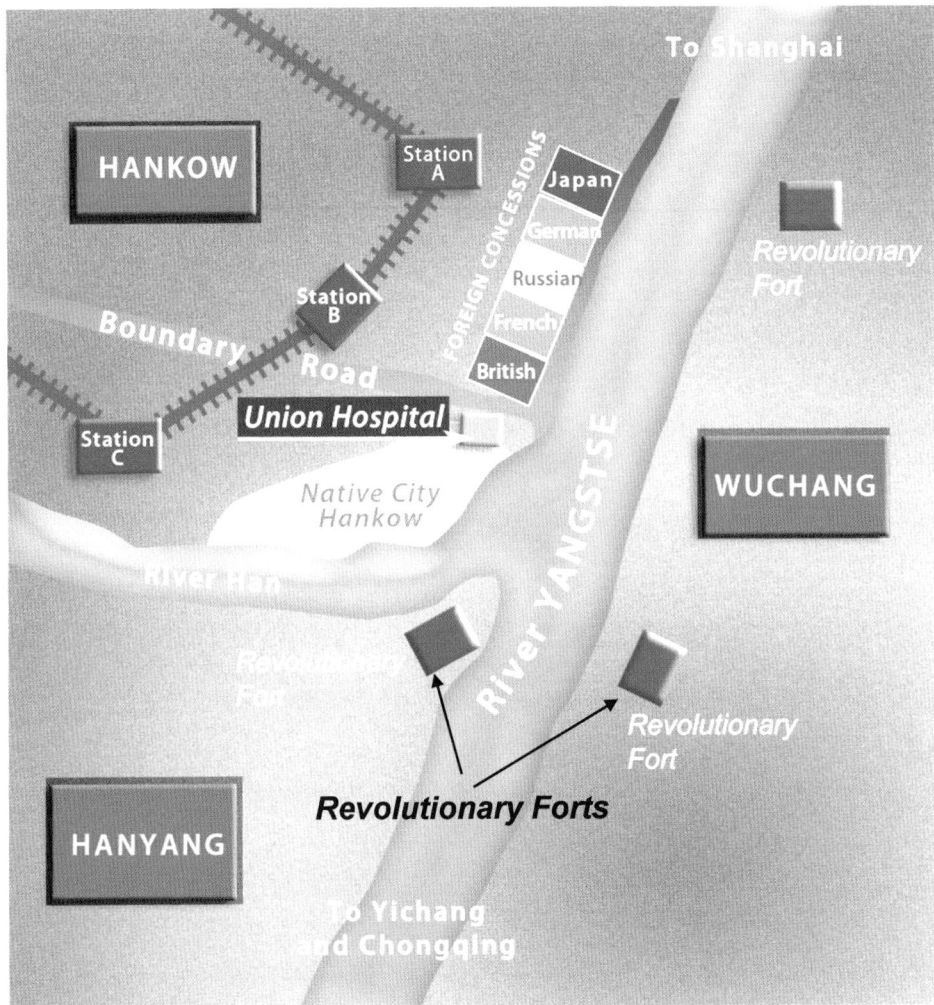

Figure 9

Outline of Imperial versus Revolutionary depositions on October 10th 1911
Illustration modified from Tom Gillison's letter to his son Walford 31/10/11

I suspect that for some reason there happened to be an abundance of sesame seed bags while the bullets were flying; normally sand bags would be cheaper. During those three hectic days of battle the Union Hospital staff members, including Tom Gillison, were eye-witnesses to the birth of the revolution which destroyed the Imperial rule and gave birth to the Republic of China.

Below is an illustration by Bessie Gillison's sister Mary Harris of the typical hairstyle and dress of supporters of the Manchu dynasty. Any male not showing a tail or "queue" was assumed to be a republican and therefore in danger of being killed during the conflict.

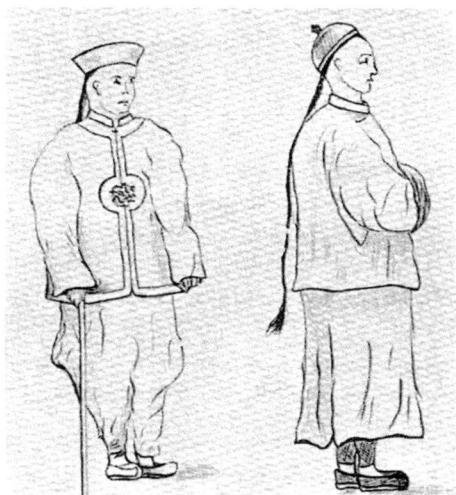

Figure 10

Chinese policeman and passer-by wearing queues which denoted loyalty to the Emperor of China
(Sketch by Mary Harris, Bessie Gillison's sister)

History relates that although the Emperor's forces won those initial battles in 1911, further engagements by the Republic forces under Sun Yat Sen won in the end. The Emperor and Imperial entourage were dismissed from Peking (Beijing) in 1912.

CHAPTER 2

EARLY REPUBLICAN DAYS (1912-1931)

In 1912 Tom Gillison and Percy McAll realised that the practice of good medicine in one isolated part of China would make only a small impact on the future health of the whole country. It was agreed by many of the missionary societies there was a great need for a larger Medical School to train Chinese doctors for the future. Following discussions with various missionary headquarters in London, Jinan (Tsinan) near Tianjin (figures 11 and 12) was the chosen site for a new large medical school; teaching started in 1917. Though its beginnings were very modest, it was the first medical school in China, founded before the Beijing (Peking) Union Medical College which began teaching medicine with the help of the American Rockefeller Foundation in 1921.

Both of these determined doctors knew there was work to be done in another direction: pioneers like Robert Morrison in South China had done remarkable work in creating a proper Chinese-English Dictionary from 1815 onwards; but there was no evidence of a Medical Chinese-English or English-Chinese dictionary. Percy McAll decided to stay behind in Jinan to concentrate on medical translations while Tom Gillison did similar work in Wuhan as shown in figure 16.

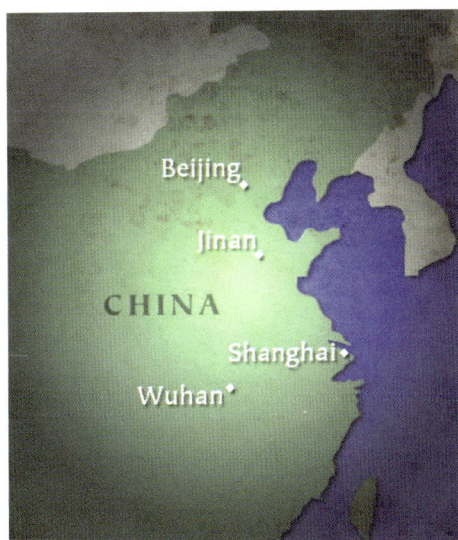

Figure 11

**Map of China showing Jinan (Tsinan)
in relation to Wuhan
and Beijing**
(Courtesy Ceri Keene)

Thus for a short period of time lasting five years the Hankou Medical School amalgamated with other embryonic Chinese medical schools to go to Jinan in 1917 to make a larger and more viable medical college, which became known then as the Quilu (Chi' Lu) University Medical College.

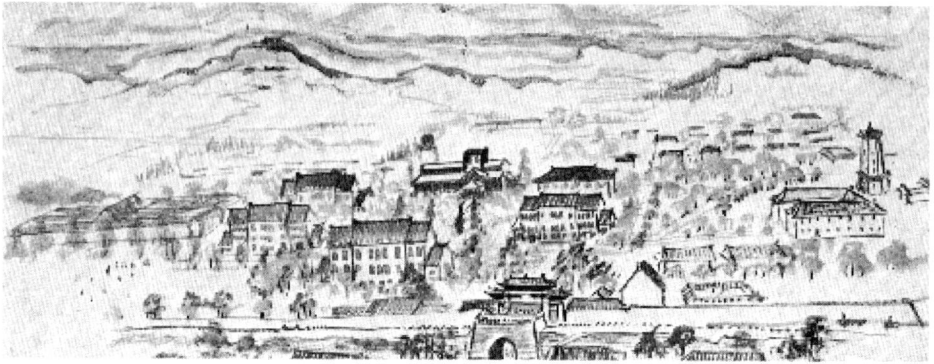

Figure 12

Quilu (Chi 'Lu) University in Jinan in North China 1941
(Sketch by Kenneth McAll son of Dr Percy McAll[14])

At last it became possible in 1923 to allow the Hubei students and staff to return to Hankou. Tom and Bessie Gillison were delighted to be able to return to where they were convinced they should spend their working lives. On his return Tom (Figure 13) was honoured by the naming of the men's wing as the "Thomas Gillison" wing. Dr Percy McAll stayed on in Jinan and finally retired there in 1935 before returning to Britain.

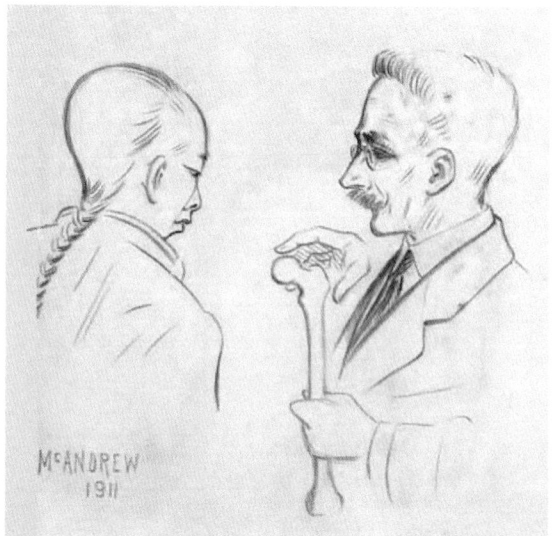

Figure 13
Tom Gillison Teaching Anatomy
"Fitting into the hip cavity it forms a powerful ball and socket joint."

16

Between the years 1923 to 1927 it was realised that the hospital premises were far too small to cope with the increasing volume of work. A vigorous campaign took place to get the funds from every possible source to build a new hospital. It should not only be larger, but it should combine male and female patients with attending staff under one roof. This would save duplication of staff, supplies and therefore cost.

Where did the money come from? This was not a state hospital but a private venture created by many different, often humble, groups of people giving amounts varying from a few cents to hundreds of dollars. Such generosity came from people not only from the city of Hankou and its surroundings, but also from centres in Britain, North America, Australia, New Zealand and other parts of the world who believed in the work and ethics of the Union Hospital. For example Tom's wife Bessie sold the house in Britain that had been given to her by her parents in order that the proceeds could be contributed towards the new medical centre. Donors like her believed that the work in Hankou was crucial for the people of Hubei who needed expert scientific help in the 20th century. In addition the London and Methodist Missionary societies each contributed £1000.00 (a lot of money in those days) towards the construction.

Thus 1928 was indeed a momentous year. It was the year the newly expanded hospital (figure 14), incorporating both the female and male wings, became the new Union Hospital and was finally built. It was a *union* in another sense of the word because it was a union of Methodist Missionary Society (MMS) medical and nursing staff with the London Missionary Society (LMS) medical and nursing staff. This huge undertaking had taken about two years of planning, fund-raising, drawing and construction to produce the finished product.

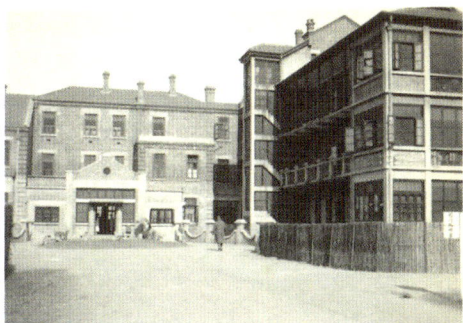

Figure 14

The new Union Hospital and main entrance completed in 1928
(Gillison family photographs)

At the time of opening the new hospital had:

1.   Five acres of land to house the buildings
2.   A main building with three storeys
3.   Six wards
4.   At the start 135 beds

In 1928[15] as many as 8455 new and old outpatients and 1171 inpatients were seen and treated. 781 operations were performed under general anaesthesia. Also in 1928 the "Union School of Nursing" was opened to provide trained nurses for the four mission hospitals in the whole of Wuhan. At the Union Hospital Gladys Stevenson was appointed matron to be assisted by Mabel Martin.

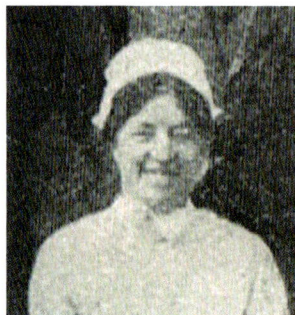

Figure 15

Portrait of Gladys Stevenson
Report of the Union Hospital, Hankou 1929

Another event took place in 1928 when the four surrounding nursing schools in Hankou were amalgamated to make one Nursing School. The first graduates in nursing were awarded their certificates the following year. At that time the Union Hospital had the largest nursing school in China.

Tom Gillison retired and Dr Edward Cundall was appointed as medical superintendent. He resigned his clinical duties and was replaced by Dr A.S. Wong. The first priority was for Tom Gillison to go back to the UK for a few months and report to the supporting churches on the medical and religious work that had taken place in Hankou. On his return to China he was determined to get down to the much needed medical translations. He said: *"I do not want to spend retirement growing vegetables in Britain, but live, work and die in China."* He got down to the task with his friend and scholar Chao Ch'i Sun (figure 16) and together they translated "Cunningham's Textbook of Human Anatomy" and "Luff's Manual of Chemistry, inorganic and organic" from English to Chinese.

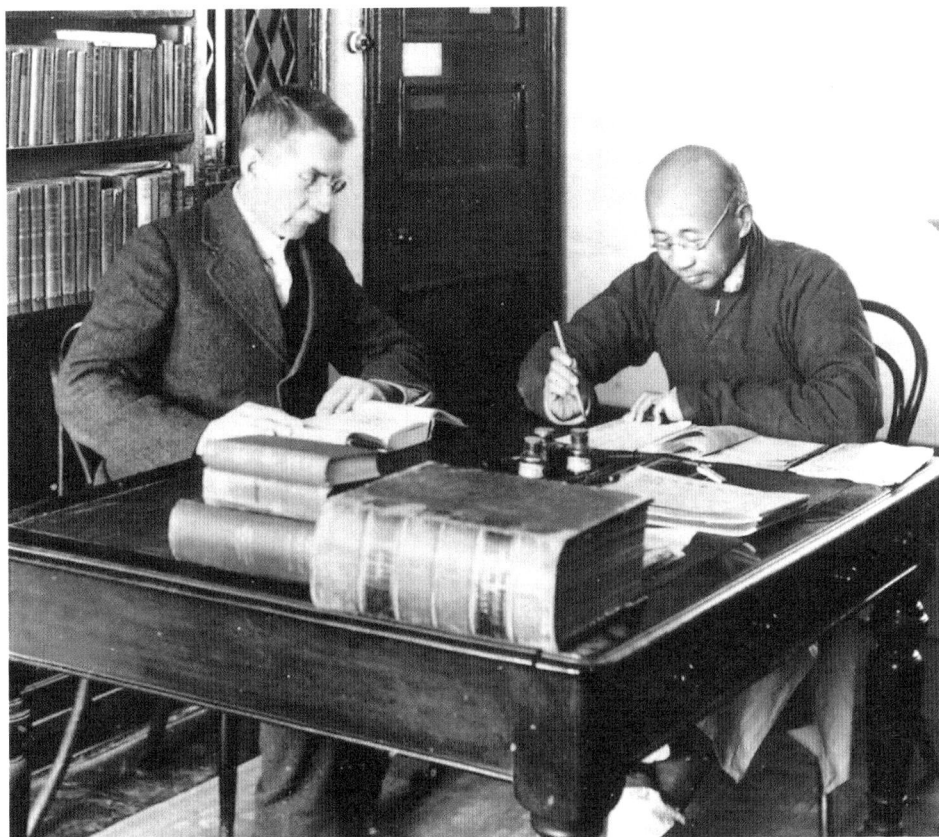

Figure 16

Tom Gillison and Scholar Chao Ch'i Sun translating medical textbooks
(Gillison family archives)

Added to all the above events in 1928, Tom Gillison's son Keith, an Edinburgh University Graduate, arrived to concentrate on surgical duties. Keith Gillison (figure 17) was a Fellow of the Royal College of Surgeons of Edinburgh, one of the oldest Colleges of Surgery in the world, which had been founded in 1504. Keith had married Kathleen Sanders in Shanghai at the end of 1927 before sailing up the Yangtse River to start working in Hankou. They both spent six months at a famous language school in Beijing before settling in Wuhan where they too believed they should live and work for the major part of their lives. Keith and Kathleen became parents to my two sisters and me; all three of us were born in China.

Figure 17

Keith Harris Gillison (1900–1988)
(Author's Collection)

In 1929 Tom Gillison's daughter Jean arrived to join the nursing staff. She had trained as a general nurse in Edinburgh Scotland, but on graduation she specialised in midwifery (obstetric nursing).

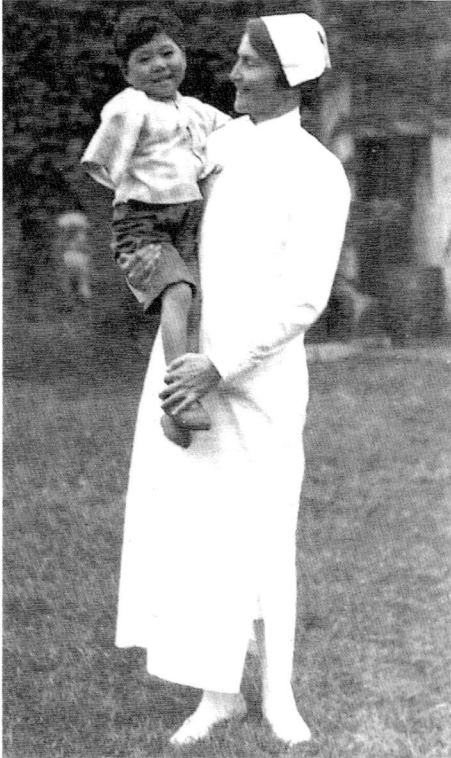

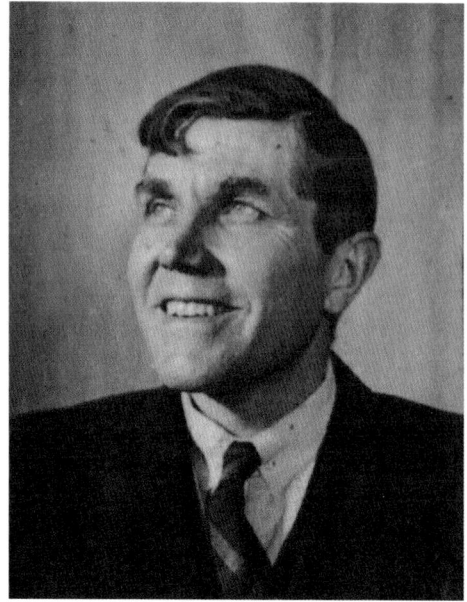

Figure 18

**Newly arrived
Nurse Jean Gillison,
daughter of Tom Gillison**
(Gillison family photographs)

In 1929 a new faculty of Public Health Nursing was created to serve the whole of China. The Union Hospital medical and nursing personnel supported this when asked by the city authorities to help in anti-cholera immunisations. Special clinics were set up which resulted in hundreds of inoculations taking place at the Hospital's City Dispensary at the Ren Chi hospital in the centre of Hankou. In the Hospital Annual report that year the main medical foes at that time were tuberculosis, cholera and dysentery[15].

The 1929 report of the Union Hospital[15] proudly reported that the reputation of the Union Hospital had increased at the same rate as the bed occupancy. Superintendant Cundall recorded the many different ways patients arrived for treatment; though most arrived by foot or bicycle, the wealthier patients came by car and the severely ill patients by stretcher. One patient even arrived on the back of a buffalo!

Medical staff numbers expanded:

1. Dr Edward Cundall, Physician and Superintendent, included his special interest in Ophthalmology
2. Dr H Owen Chapman arrived from Australia who specialised in General Medicine and an interest in Leprosy (Hansen's disease) patients
3. Dr I.S.Hsaio a general physician arrived from Shandong
4. Dr A. S. Wong replaced Tom Gillison on the staff but specialised in Ear, Nose and throat disease
5. Keith Gillison MB, ChB, FRCS (Ed) was appointed to augment surgical services
6. Dr Hadden was by now established as head of the Institute of Hospital Technology (IHT) in charge of the pharmacy, radiology and anaesthesiology departments

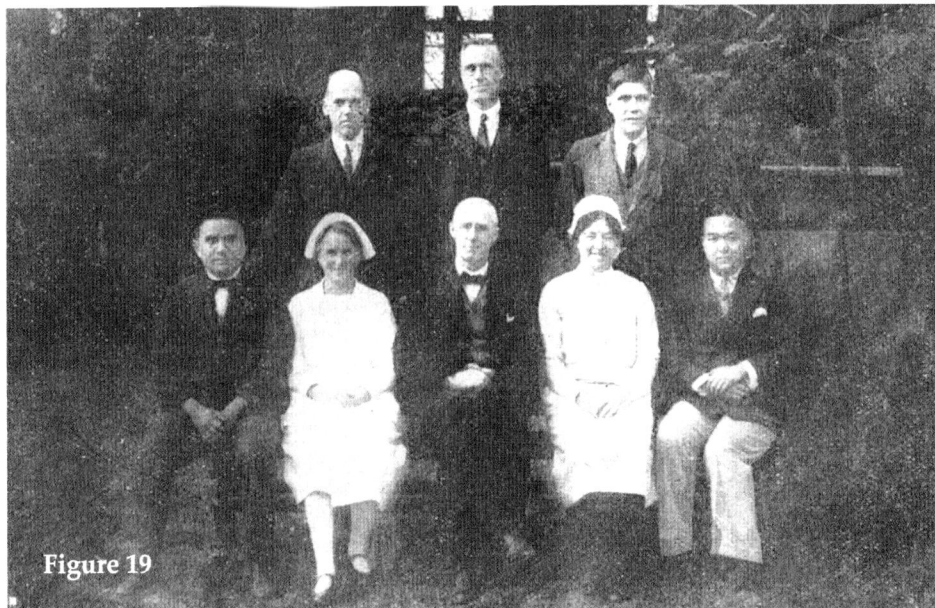

Figure 19

Hospital Staff in 1929
Back row: Dr Chapman, Dr Hadden, Dr Gillison. Front row: Dr Wang,
Sister Buchan, Dr Cundall, Matron Stephenson, Dr Hsiao
(Report of the Union Hospital, Hankou 1929)

According to Kathleen Gillison's 1929 diary there were many armed conflicts between China Communist Party (CCP) forces and the Nationalist Government mostly under the command of Jiang Jieshi (Chiang Kai Shek) in the more Northern provinces. The many soldiers from both armies who had succumbed to war injuries, especially frostbite, were admitted to the Union Hospital from those battles. The hospital made no distinction in their treatment between Nationalist Kuomintang (KMT) and CCP soldiers.

Desperately needed modern equipment was required for the new hospital. Groups such as the Ladies of Hankou Social Services campaigned and provided enough money to purchase a new steriliser. An appeal was made for funds for a badly needed X-Ray diagnostic machine because the only functioning machine in the city was in the Catholic Hospital. Previously the doctors not only had to decide the patients' fitness to travel to the Catholic Hospital, they also had to justify the expense.

At last a residential block for all doctors was opened; this meant that doctors on call were able to attend to emergencies on admission and in the wards immediately.

The figures in the 1929 report[15] showed the work had doubled since the turn of the century, although progress was occasionally impeded by illness or death amongst the medical and nursing staff. Occupancy even in the new hospital premises recorded a chronic lack of space, especially lack of beds to accommodate more inpatients. On record in 1929 there were 1492 inpatient admissions and 8415 outpatients. In those figures there were 645 inhalation and 21 spinal anaesthetics. 76 operations were carried out under local anaesthetic.

The Institute of Hospital Technology (I.H.T.) flourished thanks to the efforts of Dr Hadden and Dr Kiang, while all the para-medical services were therefore able to be provided on the hospital premises instead of being purchased from outside.

23 IHT students enrolled in the first year from 11 provinces including Korea. It was the first year that undergraduates were admitted to that faculty.

IHT facilities proudly included:

1. Laboratories in basic haematology, bacteriology and biochemistry
2. The first X-Ray machinery
3. A Pharmacy department
4. An Anaesthetic department

1930

This was a particular time of bitter civil war between Communist and Nationalist forces mostly north of Hubei. Again the hospital maintained the policy of treating all patients no matter from what political affiliation.

1930 was another hectic year for trying to keep the hospital financially solvent especially when more refugees poured in. The hospital report[16] stated a total number of 103 cases of tuberculosis diagnosed in widespread anatomical regions that had been treated. This prompted the need for an isolation ward for tuberculosis patients. That year 36 new student nurses were enrolled.

In Kathleen Gillison's diary on August 8th 1930 Keith Gillison saw his first case of anthrax infection, a disease which is still highly dangerous today. Apparently three men skinned a cow that had recently died. One of them survived but the other two showed the characteristic black spots forming a rash on their trunks; it was no surprise they died rapidly.

Just as in the previous year there were further requests for help from the Municipal Health Department in the city centres to set up vaccination and inoculation clinics. Once again the Union Hospital supplied qualified staff in support.

CHAPTER 3

1931 THE YEAR OF THE GREAT HUBEI FLOOD

1931 was a momentous year in several ways. It started off very tragically in June and July when Dr Hilda Byles (figure 7) became very ill with a severe fever. Keith Gillison was asked to see her and he aspirated some pus from her pleural cavity (chest) suspecting she had developed nasty pus around her lungs known as empyaema. He was even concerned that she might have developed a liver abscess, a well-known but highly dangerous complication. A couple of days later she had to be transferred to the International Hospital because Keith Gillison suddenly became ill from an attack of dysentery. Dr Byles got rapidly worse and died in a few days because she was far too weak for further intervention. At autopsy she was found to have a large penetrating abscess behind her heart and pericardium which was due to an empyaema following a vicious chest infection. The hospital lost a fine woman who had worked extremely hard for all the 24 years since her arrival in Hankou.

A milestone in clinical medicine was reached when Kathleen Gillison in her diary described an interesting feeding problem that arose when a man was admitted with his tongue and lower jaw (mandible) missing. He had been shot in the face by bandits because he had no money to give them. His facial wound not only looked awful but smelt awful; added to that he had not eaten for eight days. The problem was solved by having a feeding gastrostomy (a method of feeding using a fine tube inserted through the abdominal wall) under local anaesthesia so that he could be fed while his wound was treated with appropriate dressings. Though he remained quite badly disfigured, the offensive smell and discharge rapidly diminished and he soon became fit to go home.

Out of interest, the first gastrostomy was performed in Norway in 1837 for a narrowing of the gullet called oesophageal stricture in a patient starving to death. This life-saving procedure was successful and frequently used in the days before intravenous treatment of dehydration and malnutrition. Nowadays it is more popular with the benefit of fiberoptic gastroscopes allowing a feeding tube to be placed into the stomach in minutes. The Union

Hospital staff could be rightly proud of pioneering this safe, inexpensive, urgent method of nutrition in China that year.

In any part of the world where one has a huge central fertile plain nourished by a river which could swell to a mile in width in the autumn after the melting of the Himalayan snows from the west, there had always been a fear of flood disasters. The city had seemed safe from the Yangtse River after the year of 1900 thanks to the work organised by the then Governor of Hubei Province. He had constructed a 10 mile raised dyke which for 30 years had successfully contained the annual 12 metres rise and fall of the river. With that security Hankou had prospered considerably.

When the Yangtse River was higher and deeper in the autumn of 1931, on July 31st the same thirty one year-old dyke finally broke in several places. The deluge not only destroyed most of the city of Hankou but many hundreds of kilometres beyond. From that moment the water level rose steadily at the rate of about 7.5 cms an hour each and every day until it had risen about 4.5 metres (figure 20). The area in Hubei and surrounding territory, devastated by flooding, extended to a huge area of land corresponding to over 200,000 square kilometres for many weeks. (The affected area corresponded to the size of the British Isles).

This deluge immediately created over 100,000 refugees from Hankou alone who had to move quickly to higher land in Wuchang and Hanyang. Thankfully the recently built three-storied hospital had been made with good solid ferro-concrete walls and floors, so patients were temporarily safe in the upper two floors. For a few days all the staff members had to get to work by raft or boat and enter the building through the windows of the floor above ground level. On that morning of July 31st my father (Keith Gillison) told me how, while he was eating his breakfast, his feet suddenly felt cold. When he looked down he realised the coldness was due to incoming river water. By the time he got up from his chair and out of the house he had to swim the last 50 metres to reach the first floor of the patient block. All the patients had been moved by the nurses to higher floors and work continued as usual. About a week later the level rose yet another metre, so that much of the hospital was submerged in filthy water to a level 5 metres above the front entrance.

25

Life could have continued there but for the arrival of fierce storms which had caused huge wooden beams from destroyed houses to act as battering rams on all sides of the building. In his biography[17] Keith Gillison was impressed with the nurses' fortitude in their care for the patients under difficult circumstances; he was highly amused how they augmented their diet by fishing from the hospital staircases when they were off duty!

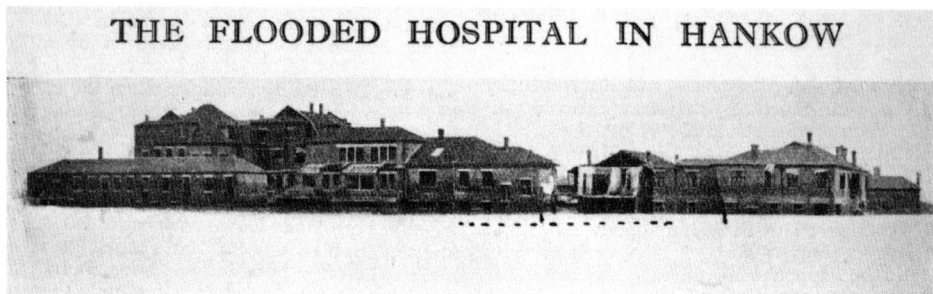

THE FLOODED HOSPITAL IN HANKOW

Figure 20

The dotted line shows one damaged end of the old Women's hospital which is seen in closer detail in figure 21
(Gillison Family Photographs)

After one such storm the relics of the "Margaret John Women's Hospital" were irreparably damaged, so it was decided that all the patients, staff and supplies had to be moved to higher ground as soon as possible.

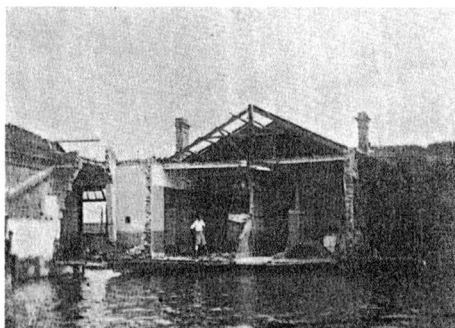

Figure 21

The old (Margaret John) Women's Hospital largely destroyed by torrents of flood water 1931
(Gillison Family Archives)

Figure 22 showed damage to the old Men's hospital as well which had been caused by wind-driven driftwood and tidal water.

Figure 22

Men's Service block failed to survive and about to collapse 1931
(Gillison Family photographs)

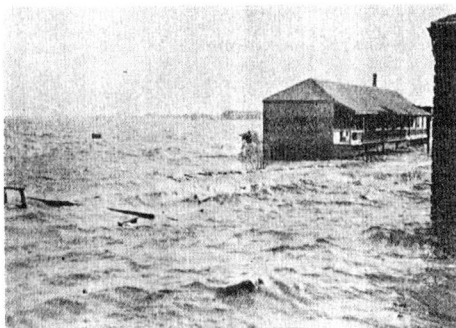

Meanwhile similar devastation had occurred throughout the rest of Hankou and the city of Wuhan. Figure 23 shows how the famous Hong Kong and Shanghai Bank had been partially submerged.

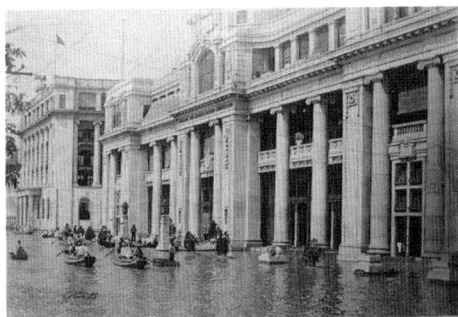

Figure 23

Hong Kong and Shanghai Bank partially submerged by floods in August 1931
YANGTSE WATER RESOURCES
COMMISSION 2001: 1931

As the newly constructed Union Hospital could not be used while it was under several metres of flood water, interim measures were taken by the foreign community of Shanghai. It generously sent some basic medical supplies on a cargo steam ship "Hannah Moller" to Hankou. For a few weeks the ship was called the men's "Flood Emergency Hospital". This measure had a limited success until problems arose getting patients to and from the ship, especially during strong winds. Added to that many patients and even some nurses were made seasick by the ship's motion in stormy weather. For a short time all male patients were transferred to the ship while female patients were transported to the Methodist School for the Blind which was fortunately vacant. It was therefore labelled as a women's "Flood Emergency Hospital".

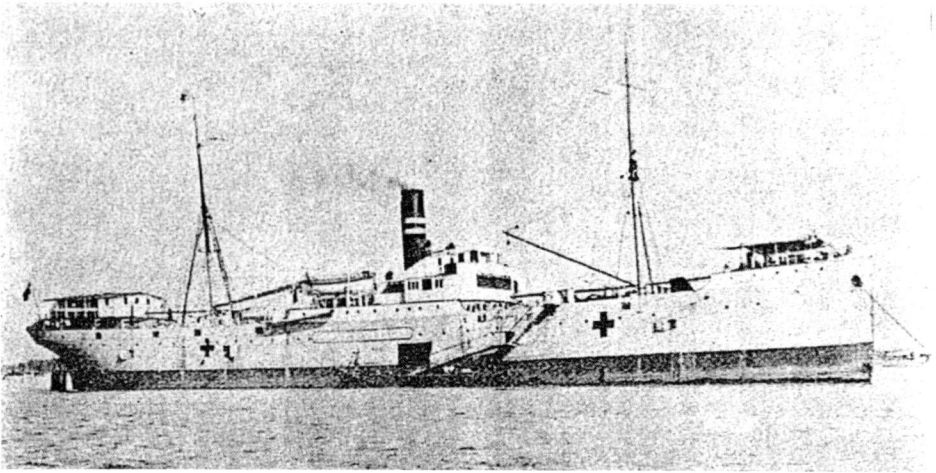

Figure 24

SS Hannah Moller acting as the "Flood Emergency Hospital"
(Gillison Photo Collection)

When the SS "Hannah Moller" was found unsuitable for patient care, the majority of male patients were transferred to the makeshift "Mat-Shed Hospital" on higher ground on Black Hill (He San) in Hanyang surrounded by 110,000 refugees. Temporary shelters were constructed by the IHT staff, some large enough to create a small operating theatre as well as serviceable wards (figure 25). All these working areas were made from poles and reed matting constructed by the resourceful Union Hospital builders and carpenters.

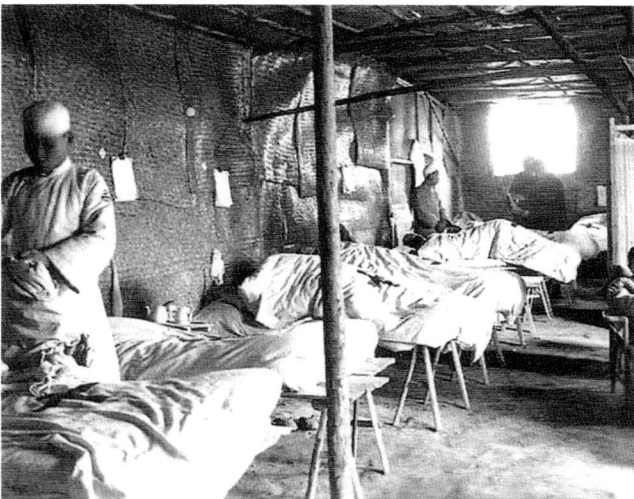

Figure 25

One of the makeshift wards in the "Mat-Shed" Hospital in Hanyang
(Gillison Family Photographs)

The moving of all patients and staff from the ship to the higher ground in Hanyang was further justified because it made access to medical care easier for the thousands of refugees as well. The floodwater persisted for approximately six months, which provided time for the much needed repairs to restore the new hospital and get it back in action.

The Mat-Shed Hospital (later known simply as the Mat-Hospital) had a reputation for giving free rice from charitable funds as well as a high standard of medical and nursing care in difficult conditions. This generosity naturally attracted more refugees from places as far away as Siaokan (Hsiao Kan) a distance of 80 miles. Unfortunately the Accounts Department noted many of those who could afford to pay, did not pay for the rice when given the opportunity. Besides them there were a huge number of refugees to care for and feed. An additional test of staff stamina according to Kathleen Gillison's 1931 diary was provided by the delivery of no fewer than 300 newborn babies in three days! Sadly many of the older children who were admitted with pneumonia were also suffering from varying degrees of malnutrition. Benevolent societies, guilds and chambers of commerce helped to keep the patients and staff alive by sending large quantities of food without charge.

It was believed that millions of lives were lost owing to the extensive flood damage over the many hundreds of square miles east of Yichang (Ichang). Back in Hanyang the City Sanitary Engineers were commissioned to build temporary shelters for toilet purposes for all the refugees gathered around the Mat Hospital. There were approximately 100,000 people estimated to be living around the Mat Hospital hospital, of which 60,000 were refugees; the Public Health problem was to find enough space between the huts to build a sufficient number of latrines. Judging by the number of recorded cases of cholera, malaria and dysentery it was a struggle. These latrines took the form of large lime pits spaced between the occupied huts; the difficulty was finding enough spaces for the latrines because of the close invasion of refugees all around.

It was no wonder cholera and dysentery infections were rife in such a close-knit community because of the shortage of latrines. There were no antibiotics in those days but the staff knew cholera killed mostly by rapid dehydration before natural germ resistance could set in. Staff members were quick to provide rapid intravenous infusions of mixed glucose and saline which saved hundreds of lives in such a time[17]. Once these patients were rehydrated, many did develop some resistance to the cholera bacterium and survived. The Union Hospital was not alone in fighting these diseases; all the hospitals in the whole province of Hubei and beyond were similarly stressed.

Needless to say great concerns were expressed about the structure of the newly built 1928 Union Hospital. How could it survive being engulfed by five metres of filthy infected Yangtse River floodwater for so many weeks? Happily when the waters eventually receded, it was obvious that while the old "Men's and Women's hospitals" were damaged beyond repair, the new "Union Hospital" (figure 14), made from strong steel and concrete girders, was more than adequate to withstand the force of those untamed flood waters. Though no one said it at the time, the money so painfully collected from so many sources during previous years had not been wasted after all.

CHAPTER 4

FLOOD RECOVERY YEARS 1931 - 1936

Elsewhere a significant event took place far away from Hubei when Japan invaded and annexed most of Manchuria, appointing the old emperor Pu Yi as a puppet figurehead (Appendix 2, the Second Sino-Japanese War). According to Kathleen Gillison's diary, news of this aggression in the north spread all over China. In Wuhan this news prompted many attempts to boycott Japanese goods. The main events during the conflict between China and Japan are summarised in that Appendix.

It was both timely and logical that the actual date the female (Margaret John Hospital) and the male (Thomas Gillison) hospital reports were formally combined was in 1932 [18].

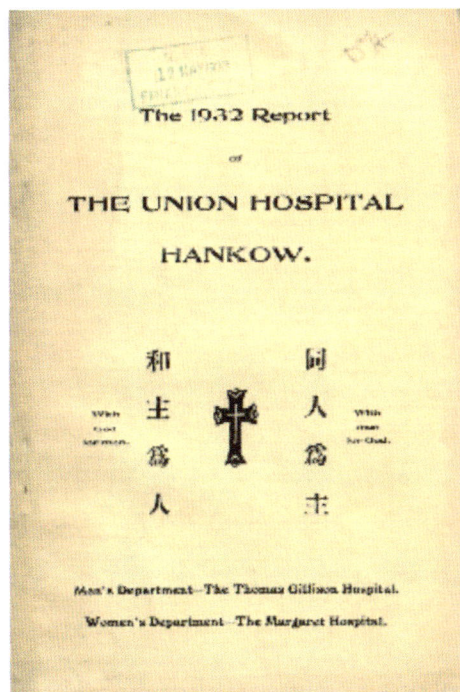

Figure 26

1932 Union Hospital report
No longer were the Men's data reported separately from the Women's "Margaret John" Hospital data

Everyone was delighted that the male patients in the Mat-Hospital, leaving the high ground of He San ("Black Hill") in Hanyang, and the female patients, leaving the premises of the Methodist School for the Blind, came back to the rebuilt hospital. For several months the new hospital was able to take advantage of all the available skilled refugee workers waiting to return to the outlying regions from whence they came.

Besides the highly infectious illnesses mentioned earlier, the physical damage of the stormy waters and the pounding effect of floating timbers had caused increased concerns for further expense. Funds from the hard pressed Provincial Government were unlikely to be available because of widespread demands for help from the whole Province of Hubei. Back in the United Kingdom the London Missionary Society and the Methodist Missionary Society campaigned for, and managed to find, extra financial support not only for the refurbishment of the hospital but also to deal with the aftermath of the floods.

Meanwhile Dr Chapman took the responsibility, with the hospital builders and carpenters, for undertaking the cleaning, repairs and reconstruction. Dr Chapman (figure 27) had been working in the Methodist General Hospital before he became senior physician at the Union Hospital. When Dr Chapman developed pleurisy for a few months, Tom Gillison came briefly out of his retirement to cover Dr Chapman's sick leave.

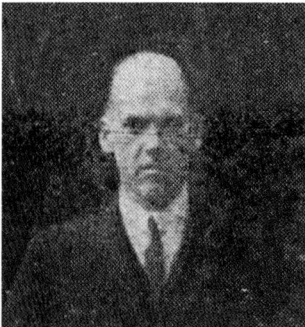

Figure 27

H O Chapman MB, DTM, Senior Physician
Report of the Union Hospital, Hankou 1929

When all the excitement and upheaval caused by the flood was over, there were changes in the medical staff of the hospital. Dr Ralph Bolton from the Methodist General Hospital provided temporary cover for Ophthalmology while the superintendent Dr Cundall was away on leave. Tom Gillison's youngest son, Dr Gordon Gillison (figure 28), arrived to help in the hospital. He introduced the technique of artificial pneumothorax for the treatment of pulmonary tuberculosis and expanded the use of novocaine spinal anaesthesia into hospital practice.

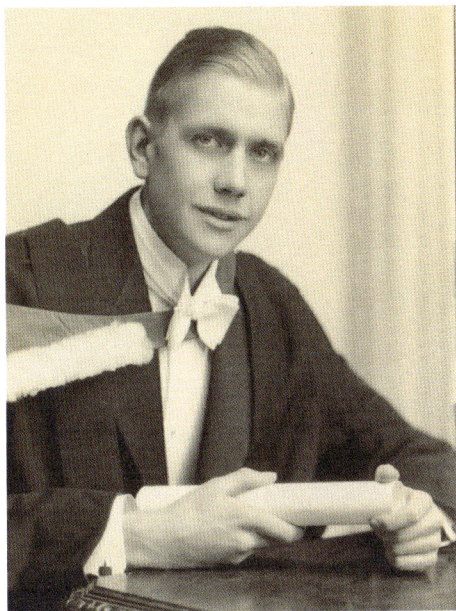

Figure 28

Gordon Colebrook Gillison
(1909 – 1941)
(Gillison Family Collection)

For the Midwifery section a 24-hour rickshaw coolie was installed to provide a 24-hour domiciliary service. It meant that the midwife on call could leave the premises at once for any obstetric emergency nearby.

1933-1935

In this year, two years after the massive floods, the restored Union Hospital not only survived but looked in a good shape (Figure 29). The compound was raised, levelled and drained which had the immediate effect of reducing the mosquito count and therefore the number of malaria admissions in the following years[19]. Medicine and Surgery became separate specialties. Inter-hospital clinical meetings with the Methodist General Hospital and other Chinese hospitals took place on a regular basis. The ratio of Chinese staff to foreign staff increased and the new "Byles Memorial" building was commissioned which improved residential accommodation on-site for the residential doctors and nurses.

Figure 29

View of the new wards built in 1929
(Gillison Photo Collection)

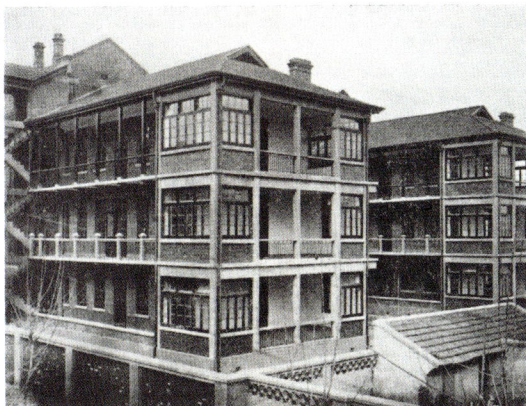

Union Hospital, Hankow, opened April 4th

Unfortunately Dr Gordon Gillison, who had been a diabetic patient since a schoolboy, succumbed to pulmonary tuberculosis soon after his arrival in China. Even today diabetes and pulmonary tuberculosis are frequent companions. With great regret he returned to the UK for rest, nourishment and fresh air in a sanatorium. That was the only treatment available in those days. He died from tuberculosis nine years later in 1941.

In 1934 a few private wards were introduced to improve income to pay towards the costs for the majority who needed free treatment[20]. This practice had been disapproved of by Griffith John some fifty-one years previously when he fell out with Dr Mawbey on that subject! However all the hospital staff by this time realised that any income from all legal sources was absolutely essential for survival. Money made in this way was used to support those patients who had severe medical and social problems but no money. It was called the "Good Samaritan" fund, the name taken from the story in the Christian New Testament. Hot water was piped on to all the wards for the first time, which made life for both patients and nurses easier and safer. The X-ray department became very much busier but it was working well.

At an international medical meeting in Nanjing (Nanking), discussions were held on the numerous medical problems in Hubei. Opium addiction was the most outstanding problem in 1934; it was commented in Kathleen Gillison's diary that there were no fewer than 56 opium dens in Hankou alone. Griffith John was still living, working and preaching around Hankou and his public statement is shown in the Opium War appendix.

Fewer Chloroform anaesthetics were given, but more regional blocks and spinal anaesthetics were used which were known to be safer and cheaper for routine operations. Dr CT Chang became a very competent anaesthetist with an expertise in providing pain relief. My father Keith Gillison confirmed that at one time two millilitres of spinal novocaine worked out to be a lot cheaper, and probably safer, for some very sick patients rather than a standard inhalation anaesthetic. He also described the possibility of layered infiltration of diluted local anaesthetic for patients with severe lung disease thus enabling a major stomach operation with a chance of a good outcome, combined with patient co-operation. When he described this operation to me many years later, this "Union Hospital procedure" inspired me to use exactly the same technique for a severe bronchitic patient with duodenal ulcer disease fifty years later in the UK. One thing I forgot was that the diaphragm immediately above the stomach has a separate sensory nerve supply in common with the same nerves that record sensation from the shoulder (cervical nerves from the third, fourth and fifth segments). During my operation the patient felt an irritation around the left shoulder caused by my touching his diaphragm. This made my patient want to bring his arm across my sterile operative field to scratch his shoulder. Once we in the operating theatre realised this situation we were able to finish the operation after pouring a few drops of local anaesthetic agent onto the surface of the diaphragm. I should have listened to my father more carefully!

The establishment benefitted from the newly arrived Dr Kung who proved that the use of instruments (the "no touch" technique) instead of using hands, however carefully cleaned, for changing dressings on the wards actually reduced cross infection. This change in nursing technique gave the additional benefit of reduced skin damage to the nurses' hands while treating and re-dressing patients' wounds.

Another advance came when the practice of 20-day bed-rest could be abandoned for skin grafted patients. It was found they fared equally well when mobilised as outpatients, thus reducing bed cost and occupancy. The principle was recommended by an eminent surgeon in London called Dickson-Wright but later published in detail by Douglas[21] in 1936.

1935 witnessed even worse flooding from the Yangtse River than in 1931 for the city of Wuhan generally, but fortunately the new 1931 flood defences were strong enough to save the hospital.

The Chinese Government rightly attempted to register all the hospitals in China for the first time. Again the Union Hospital willingly co-operated in public health programmes such as vaccination and inoculation against a range of epidemic diseases. This produced welcome publicity for the Hospital in the city. There was a mention[22] of further co-operation with the Government in introducing Health and Baby clinics in factories and to encourage other public health measures.

A better electricity supply from a central Power Station working in the city was introduced to the hospital. This encouraged more activities by the IHT department:

1. More X-Rays films could be taken
2. Diathermy could be used in operating theatres
3. Infra-red light treatment became available for physiotherapy patients
4. Physiotherapy aids using Faradic and Galvanic treatments were now possible
5. Intravenous pyelograms (a very useful method of outlining the shape and drainage of the kidneys) and early instruments for cystoscopy were available for the first time

The annual workload in 1935[22] was:

1. 9913 outpatients
2. 3478 inpatients
3. 1010 operations

This was a significant increase on previous years. Once again it had to be said in both the Union Hospital and the Methodist General Hospital, opium addiction was still the biggest enemy to health in China.

A designated rectal clinic was created for haemorrhoids (piles) as well as for other rectal conditions such as abscess, fistula and occasional tumours. Injection sclerotherapy for haemorrhoids was introduced to the Union Hospital in 1935 enabling patients to be treated as outpatients. Regrettably there is no record of the agent used; although various iron preparations had been used since 1869. The current submucosal injections of phenol in vegetable oil were not generally known until Blanchard published his work in the United States in 1931[23]. This sclerosant might have been used in Wuhan in 1935 but it was not recorded in the report.

Lymphogranuloma Venereum (LGV) was a fascinating problem in those times. It usually presented differently in men compared with women. Men were usually seen with painful swellings in the penile and inguinal regions with complications such as false urinary passages known as fistulas, also abscesses and leg swelling known as lymphoedema. In women secondary and tertiary forms of LGV usually presented in the ano-rectal region. For women the disease often presented with chronic long ano-rectal strictures. They would have to strain at stool for many hours in their attempts to gain relief. The surgical treatment which worked in those days was a long posterior median incision right through all the layers of the anal sphincter and lower rectum producing instant gratifying relief. This unusual operation was described as a "Posterior Linear Proctotomy". Many modern surgical proctologists might be horrified by this procedure thinking it would be expected to produce permanent incontinence. The Union surgical department found incontinence was virtually unknown; though very occasionally a repeat proctotomy might be required for recurrence. This was found to be a very rewarding operation[24]. Today rectal stricture due to LGV infection is rare; it is more often found in homosexual male patients and at the time of writing the disorder responds well to the antibiotic Doxycycline.

In 1935 many military spinal casualties were admitted. The thoracic and high lumbar spinal fractures seemed to do well in those days with plaster jackets arching the patients' backs for several weeks in extension in order to prevent compression of the spinal cord.

1936

While the volume of the work increased, fortunately the staff numbers increased as well.

MEDICAL STAFF[25]:
Edward Cundall (Superintendent)
Henry Owen Chapman (Senior Physician)
Keith Gillison (Senior Surgeon)
IS Hsiao (Physician)
Muriel Garnick (Obstetrician and Gynaecologist)
SW Wang (Trainee Resident in Surgery)
SL Chao (Obstetric Trainee Resident)
Collin Robjohns (Surgeon)
YK Liu (Surgeon) who had trained at Tung Nan University
YD Shik (House physician)
CW Lee (House Surgeon)

SENIOR NURSING OFFICER
James KC Liu (Nursing Association of China)

There was an increased development of special Public Health, obstetric and baby clinics but regrettably an increase of lawsuits against the hospital continued. In view of the increased lawsuits and attempted lawsuits against the Hospital, a request to the Government was made to install an independent expert medical opinion in the hope of reducing costs to all hospitals in China. This problem was good for lawyers but seldom for the patients. I could not find any record on this proposal being answered.

1936 was also the year that Public Health Clinics in the city became a permanent fixture. Two nurses were sent to Nanking for specialised training in Public Health Nursing.

That year there were:
- 661   Operations under General anaesthetic
- 355   Operations under Spinal anaesthetic
- 367   Operations under Local anaesthesia
- 333   Operations or manipulations under no anaesthesia

That made a total 1716 operations or procedures.

CHAPTER 5

THE SECOND SINO-JAPANESE WAR 1937 – 1945

Fighting between Japan and China intensified in 1937 but in fact skirmishes had been going on since 1931. As mentioned earlier, the more outstanding events are listed in the second appendix "The Second Sino-Japanese War".

According to Kathleen Gillison's diary, the Chinese Christians and many non-Christians declared they had no quarrel with the people of Japan, only with the military leaders of that country. In her diary for the following year, while travelling through Japan to reach the UK on leave, she learned from several ordinary Japanese people that Japan at that time was essentially governed by a powerful military committee or junta. It appeared that the Emperor, with or without the elected civilian government, did not have much influence on foreign policy.

1937 was also the year of what was called "The Rape of Nanjing[26]" (Nanking). The overall commanding officer (General Iwane Matsui) who had captured the city of Nanjing on December 13th was seriously ill; the next in command (Prince Asake Yasuhiko a relative of the Emperor of Japan) was in charge. He took it on himself to conduct what is now known as "ethnic cleansing". Estimates vary, but the highest published death toll was made by Iris Chang[26] who said that approximately 300,000 troops and civilians were killed. That included thousands of unfortunate women who were cruelly raped as well as being bayoneted or shot. It took several decades after World War II before some members of more recent governments of Japan admitted to this dreadful crime against humanity. W.H. Auden, a well-known British poet then staying in Hankou, said: "*And maps can really point to places, where* life *is evil now; Nanking (Nanjing) and Dachau.*"[27]

The repercussions from the Nanjing event reached Wuhan and beyond. Kathleen Gillison wrote in her diary that news of this did get through to Hankou causing some panic, especially among the nurses. Although several nurses wanted to leave the city and escape to Free China at once, it is to their credit that the majority of the Union Hospital nurses bravely decided to stay loyal to the patients and carried on working as usual.

The National government requested the names of doctors and nurses for service at the front, but the Union Hospital declined to provide the information[28]. This reluctance to disclose the names of their staff was because of the fear that they might never return. This concern became more and more acute as the Japanese army advanced from Nanjing to Wuhan. One or two doctors, besides a few nurses, moved out of Hankou, but all the foreigners and most of the Chinese medical and nursing staff decided to keep the hospital going for as long as possible. The determination to keep the hospital running compared very favourably with many other institutions in Central China.

In January 1938 Jiang Jieshi arrived in Wuhan to set up a provisional government against the military might of Japan. This brought in a rapid influx of journalists, artists and general "hangers on" for a time. Many so-called celebrities came to observe and comment on how the Chinese government was going to resist the Japanese invasion. Among these many visitors were the journalist Agnes Smedley, who was then a famous foreign news reporter, and Norman Bethune, a passing Canadian Communist surgeon who gave his remaining services to the Chinese Communist Party (CCP) until his death in 1956. Another world famous journalist in those times, James MacManus, was there. The famous British writers and poets Auden and Isherwood also arrived hoping to witness a successful military resistance to the Japanese. However the relentless Japanese bombing continued and Jiang Jieshi, while he recognised he had enough manpower, did not have enough airpower or artillery at his disposal. Therefore he decided to retreat west and organise a guerrilla type of warfare from his new capital and base in Chongqing (Chunking) until adequate air and fire power arrived[29].

Even before the Japanese occupation, galloping inflation made it more and more difficult to provide proper wages for all levels of Chinese staff; wages were produced in larger and larger bundles of notes which were getting more worthless as each month went by. According to my father Keith Gillison there was an ironic joke in the hospital about how many wheelbarrow loads a member of staff was worth! Drastic cuts in spending to pay for the much needed staff salary raises had to be made.

Meanwhile intensive bombing carried on throughout 1937 and 1938. This was so intense that many empty premises like the one below (Figure 30) were taken over to be used as a sorting centre for fresh casualties.

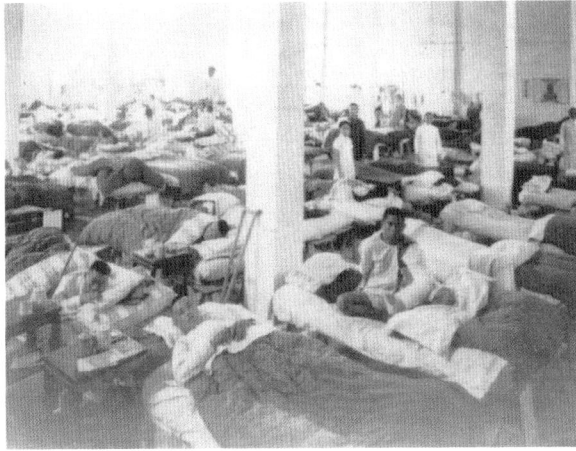

Figure 30

Temporary "Go down"
sorting centre from where
most severely injured
patients were transferred to
the Union Hospital
(Courtesy
Dr Chatterton's thesis;
p 144)

It was not unusual for Keith Gillison to examine casualties by candlelight when the power broke down again and again from the incessant bombing. According to Dr Chatterton[30] *"The Chinese nurses, having already worked during the day, returned and worked until around 3am being ready for their next day shift. When 100 more wounded were admitted, the nurses gave up their beds and slept on bamboo benches. Some of these wounded soldiers had been … lying for more than a month with very little treatment, some with limbs missing & many incapacitated for life". Clearly, and understandably, work with the wounded was exhausting and distressing".* Indeed the medical staff was very proud of the Union Hospital nurses.

Deputations from the Red Cross arrived in force, not only to give impetus to the improved co-operation between Protestant and Catholic Christians, but also to improve co-operation between Muslims and Buddhists in coping with the increased numbers of refugees. Even more refugees arrived from more eastern parts like Zhenjiang (Chinkiang), but most came from the area surrounding Wuhan as a result of the bombing.

In spite of the increased pace in the hospital work, funds for those patients who could not pay were always a source of concern. In a meeting between the International hospital and the Union Hospital on June 4th 1940 Keith Gillison was offered full time employment at the International Hospital which he politely declined even though it would have meant a salary increase. He was convinced that, like his father Tom Gillison, he had been called to work specifically at the Union Hospital. If he left he would not be able to face his friends and colleagues still working there. However he did consent to operate at the International Hospital from time to time because the individual fees provided a valuable income for the Union Hospital.

The Red Cross was able to persuade the refugees to be involved in self-help[31]: *"Chinese responsible for full time jobs in the refugee camps, such as cooks, were paid a small wage but mostly the essential work was carried out by the refugees themselves. Work was encouraged and the government funded practical industries such as sandal and towel making as well as gauze manufacture for hospital use. Under these schemes, refugees were taught to weave, provided with raw materials, portable looms and were paid. However, apart from the provision of footwear, this did not solve the immediate problem of clothing the refugees. To combat this, material was purchased to make cheap clothing produced by the local mills and from other sources"*. In addition Dr Chatterton found out that the Nationalist Government tried to help financially with the care of the thousands of refugees. In Hankou, the IRCC (International Red Cross Committee) received US $200,000.00 from the National government for the mission hospitals and all the other local hospitals attending to wounded soldiers.

Amongst all this bloodshed and damage all around Wuhan some good things emerged. For many Chinese and foreigners it was the first time that there was a sense of battling together against the common enemy of Japan[32]. *"Foreigners and Chinese endured Japanese attacks together, experiencing fear, while witnessing the after effects of air raids and artillery bombardment. Thus there developed a forging of new institutional relationships in the pre-occupation period. This was a period of greater co-operation, not only between the Chinese and foreigners, but also between the missions themselves regardless of denomination."* Perhaps for the first time in China, not only Chinese and foreign relief agencies worked together, but also Protestant and Catholic missions fully co-operated.

In 1937 the Japanese forces claimed that all foreign concessions along the Yangtse River would be spared from bombing. These areas were labelled "safe areas" or "safety zones" so the Union and two other hospitals temporarily relocated to the area of foreign concessions already shown in figure 2.[33] *"The Pu'ai (Methodist Hospital) moved from its site in the heart of the Chinese city to the Bank of China building in the previous British Concession, the Union Hospital relocated to the Salt Bank and, from Wuchang, the Methodist*

General moved to the All Saints' compound in the former German Concession in Hankou. This left the LMS Ren Chi Hospital in Wuchang, under the management of Dr. Yeh". This move was not for long because of the speed of the Japanese arrival in Wuhan.

Japanese troops entered north-eastern Hankou on October 25th and on the next day 26 vessels of the Japanese navy arrived by the Yangtse River into the centre of the city of Wuhan. As a result the city of Hanyang was taken the next day; on the 26th by land and by the river very quickly. This capitulation did at least spare more citizen casualties in Hanyang. However, in the surrounding countryside guerrilla-type skirmishes continued to be fought right up to the spring of 1945. At last the intensive bombing had stopped. The capture of Wuhan gave some advantage to the three main hospitals (Union, Pu'ai and the Methodist General Hospitals) because patients and staff could move out of the cramped conditions in the "safe areas" and continue working in their original premises.

Once again the Union and Methodist General Hospitals were surrounded by thousands of refugees because of the bombing. The hospitals were seriously deprived of the normal influx of capital from local businesses and private patients, so everyone was desperate for funds. Requests were sent out all over the Western world for financial support. One source came from the Lord Mayor of London's annual charity appeal. Records do not show how much was received but it must have been quite generous judging by a letter sent jointly by Dr Cundall of the Union Hospital and Dr Bolton of the Methodist General Hospital to the British Medical Journal in January 1938.

January 1938

Sir,

The two Hankou hospitals of British Foundation (The Union and Methodist General) although obliged to move, have never ceased to work through these critical times and are now back in their original premises working to capacity.
Through the International Red Cross these two hospitals have received money (in Pounds Sterling) for drugs and appliances. Without this help they would have been obliged many months ago to close down. This would have left the enormous

43

refugee area with no available hospital service whatever. The International Red Cross has paid a subsidy of five pence per day per bed for inpatients and one penny per visit for outpatients. The most rigid economy is practised and only patients who are really refugees in acute distress are supported by these payments.

At the time of writing the local situation is somewhat better, a little business is starting and a slowly growing population of our patients are now paying their own fees.

As some of the funds of the International Red Cross and much of its medicines and instruments were contributed through the Lord Mayor's Fund, we wish to offer our sincere thanks to our professional brothers who have helped by their generous support of the Lord Mayor's Appeal to make it possible for the institutions that we represent to continue to serve the poor and destitute at this time of tragedy.

We are etc.

Edward Cundall (Union Hospital)
Ralph Bolton (Methodist General Hospital) [34]

(In those days 240 pence or pennies were equal to £1.00 UK sterling).

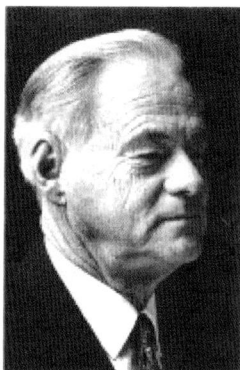

Figure 31

Collin Robjohns in later life
Portrait provided by his daughter
Margaret Howe (née Robjohns)

Collin Robjohns, a young Australian doctor with surgical experience joined the staff and was much appreciated in view of the increasing surgical work going on. Collin arrived at Union Hospital in 1935 to get acclimatised to the work and improve his language skills. He volunteered to superintend the smaller hospital in Zaoshi (Tsaoshih) for several years. He and his family were sent to Ash Camp during the Japanese occupation.

Collin's wife sadly died in captivity so Collin Robjohns returned to Australia to make a home for his daughters. He became a pioneer in a newly emerging branch of Medicine called Geriatrics which is now correctly called "Care of the Elderly".

LIFE IN HANKOU UNDER JAPANESE OCCUPATION.

Foreign medical and nursing staffs were able to continue their duties with their Chinese colleagues, but even the new Japanese-approved currency did not make any improvement in the problems of keeping the finances of the hospital stable, whether in the feeding of patients or payment of staff salaries. Japan was not yet at war with Britain or the United States in 1938 but the Japanese authorities were far from pleased to see the foreign staff carrying on working with the Chinese staff exactly as before. The continued working by foreigners was correctly interpreted as taking the side of China against Japan[32]. From the Chinese point of view this increased a sense of togetherness because all foreigners, especially in hospitals like the Union Hospital, were in the same predicament.

In 1938 staff members were pleased to welcome back Dr Cundall, who had contemplated retirement, to help until a new physician arrived. Eventually Hugh Chapman arrived from Australia to relieve Dr Cundall who was able to return to the UK in 1940.

There is no doubt the majority of the surgical work in the autumn of 1938 was increased by the fighting between opposing troops, but admissions were also increased by the many civilian casualties from the bombing which preceded the Japanese advance. Six years later it was to be the turn of Jiang and the American allies to bomb the city because of Japanese military bases dug in and around that area.

Although the Surgical department was aware of the Winnet-Orr[35] treatment of compound fractures since 1934, the increased fighting since the Japanese invasion produced a vast influx of compound fractures of all limbs, especially forearm fractures, which were not as easy to stabilise as fractures elsewhere. By definition all these compound fractures were contaminated before they reached the hospital in those pre-antibiotic days. The old conventional treatment after débridement consisted of painful repeated

45

changes of dressings, long-term inpatient care, slow healing and, on several occasions, amputation or deformity.

About this time the Union Hospital surgical staff was able to replicate the successful work on war injuries by the veteran U.S. army surgeon H. Winnett Orr.

These were Dr Orr's principles:
1. Evacuation of pus on arrival
2. Removal of any floating dead bone fragments called sequestra
3. Cleaning with standard Carrel-Dakin solution (6% bleach)
4. Packing of the wound cavity with Vaseline gauze to allow pus or serum to exit the wound freely at all times.
   This usually was associated with an offensive smell in early stages, especially in the roasting summer months.
5. Immobilisation with a partial or gutter type of Plaster of Paris
6. Added traction using pins above and below the fracture if necessary for better stabilisation
7. Finally, a review of every fractured limb after three weeks in most cases as outpatients

The IHT (Institute of Hospital Technology) department devised a comfortable and inexpensive way of immobilising these very difficult compound arm fractures using cheap, light aluminium splints to support the damaged limbs. These made the patients comfortable and the fracture sites accessible for the Winnett-Orr treatment.

Figure 32 shows the splint before being applied to the patient, showing good support around the chest with the armrest pointing out in a most comfortable angle to support the damaged limb.

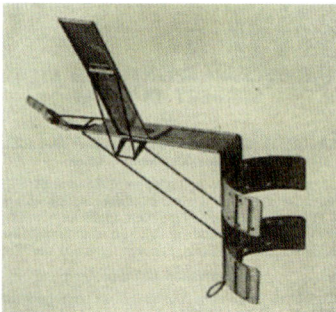

Figure 32

Abduction splint before application
(British Medical Journal 1940,
1. 686-691)

Figure 33 shows how the splint was applied to the patient providing a light and comfortable arm support while the process of healing could take place.

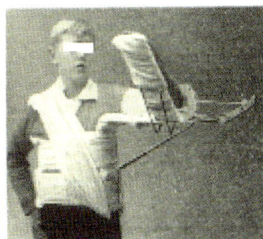

Figure 33

Abduction splint on a model showing how it was applied
(British Medical Journal 1940, **1**. 686-691)

The surgical department of the Union Hospital was able to confirm these principles worked. Despite the associated foul smell from the fracture sites, healing was surprisingly rapid. Once the fractures were clean and the bones united they could be treated either by skin grafting, further fixation with external pins or simple protection by a complete Plaster of Paris cast if necessary. This treatment was published in the British Medical Journal in 1940[36] and must surely be the first medical publication by the Union Hospital in a foreign medical journal.

Figure 34 shows an example of eleven soldiers receiving outpatient treatment at the Union Hospital for compound limb fractures just before the Japanese occupation. All eleven of them were fully mobile and comfortable with their arms in these light abduction splints while the drained and infected limbs were given a chance to heal by second intention. None of those eleven failed to heal and none required amputation; a great achievement in those pre-antibiotic days.

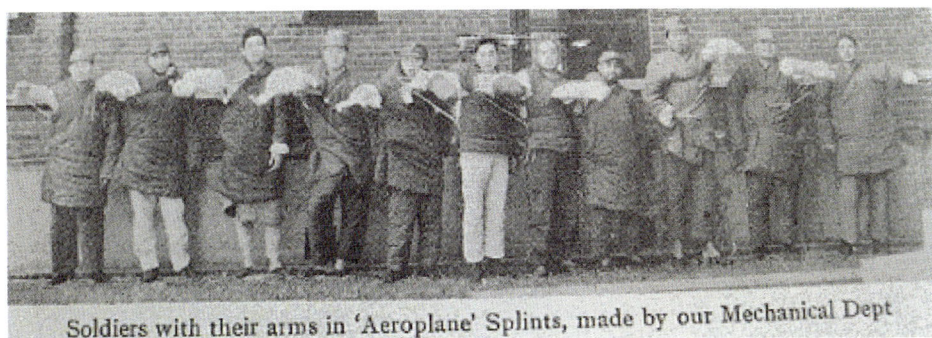

Soldiers with their arms in 'Aeroplane' Splints, made by our Mechanical Dept

Figure 34

Eleven ambulant soldiers supported by the IHT abduction splints in the Union Hospital
(Gillison Photo Collection)

Inter-hospital co-operation increased following the request for Keith Gillison to operate in the Catholic Hospital for the first time. He was able to do full lists in spite of Japanese disapproval. As a result access and expertise of the well-equipped Catholic hospital X-Ray department became available for Union Hospital patients provided they were fit to travel.

The price of rice, coal, timber and electricity prices rose very sharply. To offset this all staff (Chinese and foreigners without exception) took a reduction in wages. The financial situation was so desperate that both London and Methodist missionary headquarters responded by sending extra contributions to try to keep the hospital solvent as long as possible. Besides Japanese occupation and shortage of basic food and materials, galloping inflation became the greatest threat to survival. The Japanese introduced their "Military yen" which was used reluctantly in cities, but seldom used in the surrounding countryside

Dr Chatterton noted at around that time[37]: *"Utility supply problems persisted in Hankou but the Union Hospital was still operating with an inadequate electricity supply in 1940 despite requests through every conceivable channel…"* An *electricity generator was procured to operate the X-ray machine but this met with problems when petrol ran short. Kerosene provided fuel for lighting, but after the price tripled, the hospital changed to vegetable oil and operated a type of "mediaeval rush-lamp" for lighting. Kerosene normally $4–$5 per container rose ten-fold to $40–$60. Similarly coal, which pre-war was $20–$30 a ton rose to $200–$400 or more by the end of 1940".*

Across the world there is a saying that "Necessity is the Mother of Invention". This was absolutely true about the resourcefulness of the staff of the Union Hospital[38]:

The raw material to make Plaster of Paris was from a substance called "Gypsum Fibrosum" which was mined not too far from Wuhan. Someone in the hospital laboratory experimented with that raw material and made a suitable substance for patients who had sustained limb fractures. Likewise locally grown opium had to be harnessed to relieve patients' post-operative pain*.

Although the Battle of Wuhan was lost in military terms, that battle had an enormous influence on military progress, or lack of progress, by Japan for the rest of the war. Though there had been 225,000 military and civilian

Chinese casualties in the Battle of Wuhan, at the same time there had been 107,000 Japanese casualties. The Battle of Wuhan not only considerably weakened the Japanese Army in China; it deprived Japan of critical reinforcements in its bitter fighting against the United States in the Pacific particularly towards the end of the war.

1940

Meanwhile work carried on despite all the difficulties. Dr Chapman was now hospital superintendent with Dr YK Liu as Deputy. Dr Liu had been a house surgeon in 1937, but in the following three years he was found to be a very talented and competent surgeon, so he took on more surgical duties allowing my father Keith Gillison more time for the many administrative problems.

In this last report[39] before the closure of the Union Hospital by Japan there were the following statistics:

INPATIENTS

Total admissions	3558
Average daily occupancy	151
Average number of patients totally treated free of charge	41.8
Operations	1098
Hospital confinements	689
Home confinements	Unknown

OUTPATIENTS

Union Hospital	3419
Town Branch (Ren Chi Hospital)	1399
Antenatal patients	1907
Welfare consultations	173
Total:	11094

Inflation was so severe this particular year that salaries had to be increased more than once, with further attempts at reducing costs. Some welcome revenue came from surgical operations performed in the Catholic and International Hospitals before all foreigners were expelled in 1942. Circumstances forced Keith Gillison to spend even more time in administration thanks to Dr Liu's increased expertise and experience.

Cases of interest that year included a Chinese patient with gallstones (a condition which was more usually found in the foreign patients), patellectomy for a comminuted fracture, 12 Posterior Linear Proctotomies for LGV and the rare opportunity for a curative total hysterectomy for carcinoma of the cervix. This common operation today was a rarity in 1940 because so many patients with this disease presented far too late for surgical cure.

In 1940 the City Electrical Power Station had been destroyed by Japanese bombing; therefore the hospital petrol-driven power generator was conserved for X-Rays and operating theatre lighting. To save this precious fuel, oil lamp lighting was further used on the wards after nightfall. By this time petrol had become more expensive as a result of inflation[37]; it had to be used as sparingly as possible.

Because at first Japanese troops were temporarily billeted under canvass in the park next-door to the Union Hospital, many outpatients found it preferable to be seen in the Ren Chi Town branch, though eventually more got through to the Union premises as time went by.

CHAPTER 6

GLOBAL WORLD WAR 1941 – 1945

Japan's "New Order for East Asia"

On December 7th and 8th 1941 Japan declared total war on the United States and Britain by the simultaneous attacks on Pearl Harbor and Hong Kong. Almost in minutes, Japanese officers arrived at the Hospital premises where all the British staff members were informed that they and all the other British residents of Hankou were to attend a meeting with the Japanese Garrison Commander. At this meeting it was announced that because Japan was at war with Britain all enemy subjects were to be confined to their homes. The very same day Japanese soldiers arrived at foreigners' homes to confiscate cameras and wireless sets (radios). All foreigners who were now enemies of Japan were told to await further instructions.

Back at the hospital in 1941 bread supplies continued by organising local flour mills to deliver grain directly to two store rooms on the hospital site. It may have taken three hard-working men, a blind pony and a donkey to grind the flour, but the patients did somehow get fed!

Before all the commercial business closed or moved west, some private income was generated to keep services going. To everyone's surprise 1152 operations had been completed. The hospital was pleased as well as surprised that the number of operations completed in 1941 was greater than in 1940 (1098 operations).

At the end of 1941 the Union Hospital funds were again rapidly running out. This was because:

1. Incoming funds from the usual local and foreign business companies had diminished since key personnel had left the city
2. Wards had to be closed due to staff shortages and diminished food supplies
3. By now very few patients capable of paying for treatment were living in Wuhan who would normally contribute financially

Credit must be given to the Australian Senior Physician Hugh Chapman (figure 27) who had somehow got access to funds from his friends and relatives in Australia. He took over the post of Superintendent, releasing Keith Gillison to help in the busy Surgical Department. With great skill Dr Chapman kept these funds away from the prying eyes of the Japanese and their few Chinese sympathisers. No doubt in the same eyes of the Japanese administration this measure was illegal, but it meant that this money, with an added generous loan from a local Chinese well wisher (who was repaid in 1942), somehow kept the hospital financially solvent at a crucial time. This clandestine account was called "The Hospital Stores Account" and was never discovered[40].

The banning of public meetings and the difficulty in obtaining passes gave Superintendent Chapman greater local responsibility. It was very fortunate he had worked closely with Dr YK Liu who would eventually take over once all foreigners had been expelled. It was soon made clear that all foreign enemies of Japan were either to be repatriated in exchange for Japanese Prisoners of War (POWs) or go into internment camps near Shanghai.

For a short while the medical work continued as before. This tougher and more restricted climate produced a much firmer bond between the foreign and Chinese colleagues. Foreign citizens had to wear bright red armbands (Figure 35). "A" denoted American citizens and "B" for British citizens etc, so that the Japanese military could keep a check on all foreign personnel moving around the city. Keith Gillison being a British citizen had to have a special pass as well as wear his armband every Tuesday when he crossed the ferry across the Yangtse River to his regular Wuchang clinic.

Figure 35

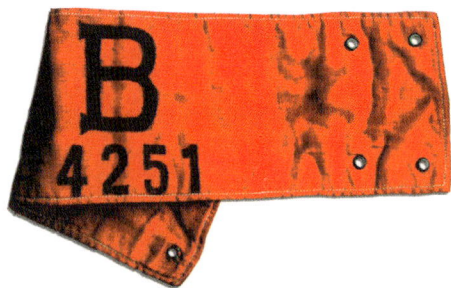

Typical armband for British citizens to be worn outside the Hospital at all times
(I am indebted to Greg Leck for permission to publish this image from "Captives of Empire") [41].

In Hankou, once the foreign staff had been sent to Shanghai for repatriation or Internment camps, Japanese Army officers made more frequent visits to the Union Hospital, which raised the fear that the Japanese military was going to take it over. This fear was realised later when the Japanese Army Medical Service arrived. These new arrivals announced the hospital was to be used exclusively for Japanese patients as a fever hospital. It was to be staffed by Japanese doctors with Japanese and Korean nurses working in Central China. It was made clear that all Chinese personnel, whether patient, medical, nursing or technical staff, had to leave the Union Hospital premises immediately. Fortunately the IHT staff had already anticipated this might happen; they had already moved themselves and much of the equipment to Free China.

The expulsion of the chronically ill patients was particular distressing for patients suffering from Leprosy (Hansen's disease). Leprosy then required long term medical and drug treatment. Dr Chapman had a special interest in Hansen's disease and feared these patients would not survive.

Having taken over the Union Hospital, Japanese attention was turned to the Ren Chi branch of the Union Hospital. Interference was warded off by Dr YK Liu who had shrewdly invited Wuchang's mayor (a Japanese sympathiser) to make a personal visit and become nominal president. While the Ren Chi branch had excellent outpatient facilities, it did not have anything like enough space for inpatient care, particularly for the displaced Union Hospital inpatients.

On August 12th 1942 Dr Y.K. Liu officially became senior surgeon as well as hospital superintendent after Hugh Chapman's departure for the Lungwha internment camp in Shanghai. He transferred every patient with as much precious equipment and drugs as he could possibly salvage to the empty Young Women's Christian Association (YWCA) quarters in the City centre. This makeshift building was named the "Ho Chi Hospital". Instead of 240 Union Hospital beds, Dr Liu had to manage as best he could with only about 100. His Physician colleague Prof Ye, father of Prof Ye Professor of Gynaecology in recent years (see dedication), was of tremendous help, not only for his professional services but by acquiring expert assistance from a Mr SP Li acting as business manager.

Dr Liu demonstrated impressive skills of leadership:

1. He had successfully resisted the threat of a Japanese takeover of the Ho Chi Hospital by appointing the local mayor as president, known for his approval by the Japanese. This manoeuvre protected both the Ren Chi and the Ho Chi hospitals.
2. Where he found any sign of corruption such as theft of precious hospital supplies, he dismissed those perpetrators even though some of them had the skills that he would have liked to retain. He wanted to show the world a "clean sheet".
3. He managed to keep the hospital functioning along the teaching hospital principles of training doctors and nurses as well as caring for patients. The Nursing School continued to train more nurses despite the difficulties under enemy occupation.
4. He managed to keep the hospital solvent for two years with revenue only coming from patients and local community. To his surprise some of the revenue came from a few residual private patients; a remarkable achievement in a very frugal environment.

In later years this whole move was perfectly described by the returning Dr Chapman as follows[42]:

"Dr. Liu had shown unsuspected reserves of strength, proving equal to every demand that was made on him. He took entire control of the new hospital under a Supervisory Committee appointed by the two local church bodies representing the Founders [LMS and MMS]. Though threatened by both Japanese and Chinese racketeers, he stood firm. . . . Dr Liu met all potential disasters and the occupiers with that mixture of patience, tact, compromise and firmness of which so many Chinese are past masters."

It is no exaggeration that this Dr Liu was the saviour of the hospital itself when otherwise the whole institution could well have collapsed in 1943. As author of this book I deeply regret I cannot find a portrait of this remarkable man.

In the continued spirit of co-operation never seen before the Japanese occupation, the Roman Catholic Hospital shared its laboratory services for testing for malaria while the Union Hospital shared its very experienced midwifery services before and after the take-over. Both hospitals benefitted enormously in such very difficult times.

By the end of 1942 all enemy foreigners had left Hankou. While many had hopes of repatriation in exchange for Japanese prisoners of war, in actual fact the majority were sent to civilian internment camps mainly near Shanghai. Keith Gillison and his family were sent to Yangzhou (Yangchow) on the Grand Canal about 200 miles from Shanghai shown in figure 36. Dr and Mrs Chapman went to Lungwha, Dr Collin Robjohns to Ash Camp in Shanghai and Nurse Jean Gillison went to the Pudong (Pootung) Prisoner of War (POW) camp.

On a happier note; between the years of 1928 to 1942 the Union Hospital had trained no fewer than 115 General Nurses who had received the national diploma of NAC (Nursing Association of China). In addition 100 qualified Midwifery nurses had been trained.

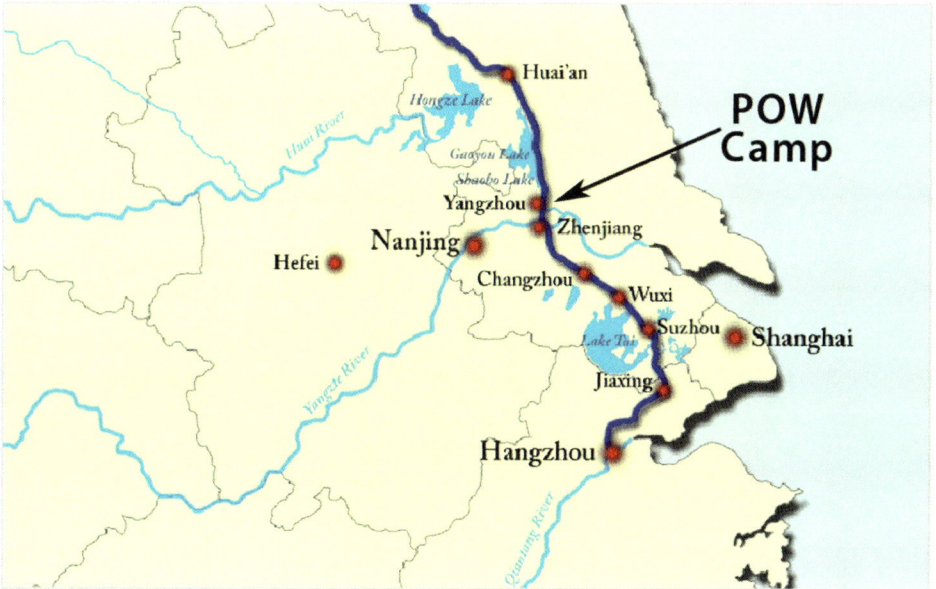

Figure 36

Location of Yangzhou on the Grand Canal 200 miles from Shanghai
(Gillison Family Collection)

Dr Chatterton confirmed the findings of others looking at other parts of China; that Japan wanted to remove Western influence in Central China for the following reasons[43]:

1. To increase security for Japan for **military** reasons. This had always been thought to be the principal explanation.

2. To expel all Western **religious** influences on the Chinese churches

3. To exclude all Western **medical** influence on Chinese hospitals.

In Japanese eyes the sooner all Allied westerners were dismissed the better.

At last in 1944 when the balance of the war turned in favour of China and her Allies, bombing from Free China took place. On December 18th American bombing, based from Chunking, destroyed large parts of the city, sadly including the Ho Chi Hospital. Staff risked their lives and their bodies to try and rescue as many of the patients that they could. There were accounts of the staff uniforms being burnt off the backs of the rescuers because they would not rest until all possible staff and patient survivors had been rescued.

Until it was flattened by the bombing, Dr Ye had managed to keep the Ho Chi Hospital financially viable throughout the war. He was helped by the quiet presence of Dr Oertel (a German national) who was unmolested because the Japanese authorities wrongly assumed him to be a supporter of the German government. It was fortunate the significance of Dr Oertel being a Jew was unknown to the Japanese in Wuhan, as between them Drs Liu, Ye and Oertel saved the hospital from a complete Japanese takeover and very possibly complete oblivion.

Records showed that Dr. Liu had remained in charge until early in 1944 when he was transferred to another hospital, leaving a new colleague Dr Wang in charge. The Ho Chi Hospital had clearly survived under Chinese leadership with no external help at all. Dr Chapman, in his 1945 report[44,] referred proudly to the Hospital's continuation under Chinese leadership as a "witness to the faith that was in it".

Meanwhile the removal from their vocations and workplaces had been very frustrating and heartbreaking for the Wuhan foreigners. For two and a half years it was impossible for them to find out what had been going on until the war was finally over. Time and time again in her 1945 diary Kathleen Gillison wrote how frustrated she and her husband Keith were by the lack of news from Wuhan.

Chapter 7

WORD WAR II AFTERMATH. 1945 to 1950

Though the war officially ended on August 15th 1945 it took several weeks for the British POWs in various internment camps to get out of captivity. For example Keith Gillison and family were unable to be released from the Yangzhou POW camp for six weeks (October 1st.) Dr Chapman and the Revd Harold Wickings were the first to travel back to Hankou in order to report back to their mission headquarters as soon as possible.

On his return Dr Chapman congratulated the whole staff of the Ho Chi Hospital which was struggling to return patients, equipment, and stores as well as personnel to the Union Hospital. They found the hospital premises were still occupied by stranded Japanese patients who had not been transported back to Shanghai and Japan with their retreating troops. Harold Wickings commented on those Japanese still left in the city[45] *"Thousands of Japanese temporarily stranded in Hankou would have liked to have had Chinese nationality and remain in Wuhan"*.

Dr Chapman also commented that the hospital staff had not only endured the Japanese occupation but also the "taunts of its friends in Free China". He said *"it was bad enough for the staff to withstand the privations of living and working under enemy occupation, but it was also an insult for those who had stayed behind being accused of collaboration with the Japanese by staff who returned from Free China"*[46]. Those who stayed understandably called themselves "Loyalists", while those who returned called themselves "Patriots". It took some time for resentments between these two groups to be reconciled after the war.

In his publication Keith Gillison[47] was thankful that although the chapel had been flattened, the main hospital structure which had been built to such a high standard in 1928 had withstood the bombing very well. This compensated to a certain degree since the Ho Chi town branch, the Catholic Hospital and the International Hospitals had all been completely destroyed by the incendiary bombing the previous year. He confirmed that several hundred Japanese fever cases needed treatment before repatriation, which caused added headaches to all the agencies trying to restore normal medical services.

In the Union Hospital premises there was a widespread mess and chaos in all departments. Most of the equipment such as the X-Ray machines had been vandalised or stolen. However help arrived from several directions: The Hospital at this crucial time was indebted to the Friends Ambulance Unit (FAU)'s relief and rehabilitation work. In early October an agreement was drawn up between the FAU and a committee of the Union Hospital Board composed of Drs. Chapman, Bolton and Gillison, Nurse Jean Gillison and the Revds. Wickings, Geddye, Griffiths, and Rees[48]. This meeting was quite an achievement as several members of the committee had only a few days before been released out of their respective POW camps. For example Keith Gillison had just arrived in Shanghai on October 2nd, six and half weeks after the armistice had been signed in Japan. It was agreed that the FAU medical team under the direction of Canadian Dr Robert McClure should re-open part of the Union hospital with a skeleton staff working with 40 inpatient beds.

There is no doubt that practical decisions like these had to be taken by people on the spot in Hankou. Such decisions carried more weight than any decisions by Missionary Societies sitting behind desks 5000 miles away in London. This remarkable co-operation between relief agencies in Hankou and London paid dividends. By accepting that agencies such as the FAU and UNRRA (United Nations Relief and Rehabilitation Agency) should be given unprecedented power to equip, repair and maintain staff salaries for six months at their expense turned out to be providential. It enabled the hospital to get to work and earn its own crucial income as soon as possible.

The Canadian Robert McClure, with much experience of working in Free China in emergency medicine, was asked to co-ordinate the centralisation of resources and the purchase of drugs and new equipment. Dr Edward Cundall, who had retired from being Superintendent before the war, returned yet again to help restore things towards normality and promised to stay for a year. A Methodist minister called the Revd JJ Heady, already living and working in Wuhan, acted as an administrator and bridge between the above Relief agencies and all the missionary authorities back in the UK.

Not only were the premises cleaned up but many of the old staff, who had fled the Japanese invasion, happily volunteered to help get the place fit for its original use. Miss Hilda Waddington a staff member of the Institute of Hospital Technology (IHT) which had been sent to Chonqing in 1938, returned with several Hankou nurses to provide a skeleton cover for inpatient care[43].

The members of staff were delighted to welcome back Andrew Chang, a very experienced nurse who had excellent radiotherapy and anaesthetic skills. Very soon there were enough new people and residual staff to care for those first 40 inpatients in premises provided at very short notice by the FAU. Dr McClure spent several months helping out in other ways, such as equipping the medical and surgical clinics while order was restored to open up the rest of the hospital. These clinics were ready and willing to start work again on December 11th 1945. This rapid action by the FAU and the relief agencies gave the foreign staff some precious time to recover from their POW experiences and come back to help keep the hospital in full active service.

In the main hospital three new diagnostic X-Ray machines, two radiotherapy machines, film processing units, film dryers, a Geiger radium detector and many other accessories arrived in a remarkably short time. Such equipment attracted paying patients who could afford modern investigations and treatment; it turned out to be providential during this period of crippling post-war inflation.

Even charitable causes outside Wuhan rose to the occasion of keeping the Union Hospital solvent[43]. For example, the ordinary citizens of Sheffield in Britain collected enough money to buy and transport to China a modern motor ambulance. From other charities came a 20 ton truck, two fine electricity generators and a water-distilling machine which could produce 60 gallons of distilled water in an hour. This item not only provided enough distilled water for the hospital, but it also generated some income to sell to other institutions in the city. As a result of these additional items of modern equipment, while other hospitals were struggling financially, the Union Hospital was able to attract more fee-paying patients and make ends meet during such an inflationary environment. These advances in activity meant the hospital bed count was able to increase quite rapidly from 40 to 240 beds within a year.

Keith Gillison came back from leave ostensibly to continue surgical work, but was again asked to act as superintendent. This was thanks to the availability of young Dr Chang Pao-Lo (Paul Chang) who was by now a very experienced and competent general surgeon. Keith Gillison was reluctant to become superintendent because he felt it was time for a Chinese doctor to take over the task of overseeing the day-to-day administration of the whole enterprise. He did so in the spirit of a caretaker superintendent. Although he had spent more than half of his life in China, he had to obtain a proper permit (Figure 37) to continue to practise medicine in the Union Hospital.

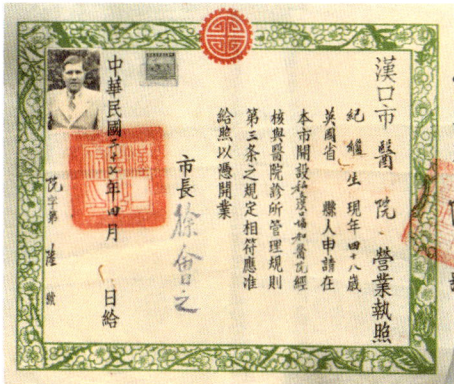

Figure 37

(Gillison Family Collection)

Translation:

Dr Gillison of 48 years of age is applying for opening the private-owned Hankou Union Hospital. The application has been checked as obedience of the third of the management rules of hospitals and clinics.

The application has been approved.

Mayor Xu Hui-Zhi (signed with a blue seal)

Republic of China, April 37th year.

This is the sixth document for the hospital application for opening.

Since Hugh Chapman, Ralph Bolton and Keith Gillison had been away, they strongly believed that the time had come to think of joining up the Union and Methodist General Hospitals with the School of Nursing and the newly established School of Midwifery to form a proper teaching hospital to train the future doctors and nurses of China. They called the organisation the provisional Central China Christian Medical Union, CCCMU.

Despite the carnage during the war, the population around Wuhan had increased and was increasing to about two million citizens. Now 50 years later the population is above 10 million people. From the health point of view it seemed intellectually and economically wrong to send major and complicated cases hundreds of miles away to Nanjing, Hong Kong, Shanghai and Beijing while there was the will, the expertise and resources to form a major academic and teaching hospital in Wuhan to provide expert services to the province of Hubei and beyond. In 1947 Senior Physician Hugh Chapman and my father Keith Gillison submitted a proposition to the Post-war Chinese Government to consider the beginning of a larger medical school in Wuhan which would train many more doctors, nurses etc in the future. The document was called "Teamwork for Health in Central China" which has been summarised in Appendix 3. The request was acknowledged but with the momentous Civil War between Jiang's Kuomintang (KMT) and Mao's Chinese Communist Party (CCP) armies this matter was put aside.

In 1949, despite much political upheaval during a year of civil war between the armies of Jiang Jieshi and Mao Zedong (Mao Tse Tung), it turned out to be another year of considerable progress for the Union Hospital.[44.]

1. The whole hospital was screened with copper mesh to reduce the ingress of flies and mosquitoes into the wards and departments

2. The first mobile X-Ray units were available to enter the wards to take diagnostic images of seriously disabled patients

3. Chloromycetin was first used for life-threatening infections with great success

4. Radiotherapy in the form of implantable needles was available and used for the treatment of cancers. Buildings made for the first proper therapeutic external beam radiotherapy machinery were installed

5. The diagnostic X-Ray department was expanded thanks to the five new machines now in action

On May 16th 1949 the city of Hankou was officially liberated by Chairman Mao's forces[47]. In spite of the upheaval the work went on as usual.

Representatives of the new government of Communist China arrived and at first discussions were very satisfactory. It was agreed for the present that the hospital should continue in exactly the same way until a permanent policy for health in the city of Hankou had been decided. An added difficulty for the medical work to continue normally was the requirement for all Chinese staff to attend political meetings during working hours on a regular basis. This made patient care on the wards and in the operating theatre very difficult. Nevertheless, staff members typically co-operated in this new environment and continued to care for patients in their usual professional manner.

Later on in the year life became increasingly difficult. Foreigners noticed that social contact between Chinese and foreign staff members was discouraged. One longstanding Chinese friend of my mother declined an invitation to a meal at home for fear of being accused of being an "Imperialist spy". About the same time the new Government passed a law saying that the proletariat was able to sue any private or non-governmental institution free-of-charge including the Union Hospital. However trivial or fictitious a charge that might be made; the Hospital had to be defended.

As Keith Gillison was superintendent and fluent in Chinese he had to spend more and more of his working hours in court defending the hospital against any and every charge that had been made. This meant that certain non-urgent operations requiring his performance, assistance or attendance had to be done out of office hours and frequently during the night.

Early in 1950 a statement came from Beijing that all foreign and Chinese Christians had five years to allow and develop complete autonomy of all mission hospitals in both the religious and medical senses. This seemed very reasonable as it was always the policy in the Union Hospital that it should be run by staff members at all levels who were Chinese. This orderly takeover was sabotaged by the advent of the Korean War which started on June 25th 1950. This new war took place between North Korea, supported by China and the Soviet Union, and South Korea, supported by Britain and the United States of America. As a result of this dramatic event the five-year agreement was scrapped and local Governments decided that all foreigners who were not members of the Communist Party should be dismissed or made to leave instantly[47]. In Hankou militant members of the staff Communist Party encouraged an organised strike against the Hospital to speed up the dismissal of all non-Communist foreigners. The strike was not unanimous and was abandoned after a few days.

By the year of 1950 the changes to the staffing of the hospital were impressive. Whereas in 1866 the hospital had started with one doctor and a couple of trained orderlies, the staff numbers had risen to:

1. 20 qualified doctors. (15 Chinese, 4 British, 1 Canadian and six interns who had just graduated from other medical schools)
2. 20 qualified nurses
3. 89 student nurses
4. 4 diagnostic radiology machines
5. 1 radio-therapeutic treatment machine for cancer
6. An Institute of Hospital Technology training anaesthetists, radiographers, laboratory technicians, pharmacists and physiotherapists qualified to work all over China.

All this had happened despite wars, revolutions, bombing and floods in that first period of eighty four years.

Back at the hospital the eminent surgeon Paul Chang not only refused to strike but also refused to give up his Christian beliefs. It was no surprise he was later ordered to serve in the new military conflict in North Korea. He was believed to have died in that conflict because he never returned to Wuhan. For his personal charisma and his surgical skills Paul Chang was badly missed[47]. Further difficulties for the foreign medical and nursing staff occurred when any conversation that did not directly involve patient care risked a Chinese colleague being accused of lacking in full support for the new Government. The foreign missionaries did not take long to realise they could be an embarrassment to their Chinese colleagues and friends; therefore it became an obvious decision for them to leave China immediately. Sadly for many of them, a return to China was not possible for the remainder of their lives.

Keith Gillison left the Union Hospital in June 1950 with great regret because all his life he felt he was destined, like his father Tom Gillison, to spend his whole life in China. Though he found plenty of work to do in the UK and years later in Nigeria, he was very sad to leave the place of his birth and where he believed he should spend his whole working life. Nevertheless, he was comforted by the fact a fine Chinese, Dr Fang, known to my parents as Yao Ker Fang (figure 38), was appointed as his successor before his departure. Dr Fang was a person with whom he had worked, whom he respected and had got to know for some time[49].

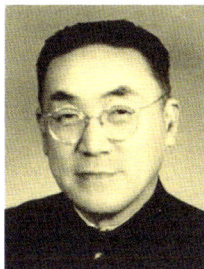

Figure 38

New Superintendent
Yao Ker Fang

(Archives Wuhan Union Hospital 1866 – 2011)

Before 1950 not all members of the hospital staff, both Chinese and foreign, were Christians. However time and time again the staff showed they were willing to give their lives, their health and their hearts to the Union Hospital. Their beliefs in the routine hospital reports regularly stated the hospital's ethos in Figure 39.

Figure 39

THE UNION HOSPITAL ETHOS IN 1866 AND IN 1950

1866

With God for men
With men for God

After 1950
"Letting a hundred flowers blossom and a hundred schools of thought contend is the policy of promoting progress in the Arts and Sciences and a flourishing socialist culture in our land."[50]

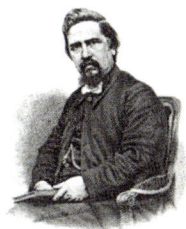

Griffith John (1831-1912)

Mao Zedong (1893-1976)

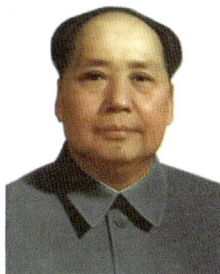

See figure 1

en.wikipedia.org/wiki/Mao_Zedong

It might appear that there was little common ground between the two ideologies. Previously the hospital was run privately through great and small sacrificial giving from local Chinese citizens and from well-wishers all over the world until the arrival of the new government in 1950. The hospital became a State institution from 1949 to 1950 onwards, yet the concern for the patients of Wuhan and the training of both doctors and nurses continued to the highest possible ethical standards as it did before the revolution.

Since 1950 when the Chinese government took over the running of the Union Hospital, all the foreign doctors and nurses took some satisfaction as well as comfort that their past efforts to contribute towards the viability of the hospital had been achieved. They wished unreservedly for the staff and the patients the best possible fame, fortune and health in the future.

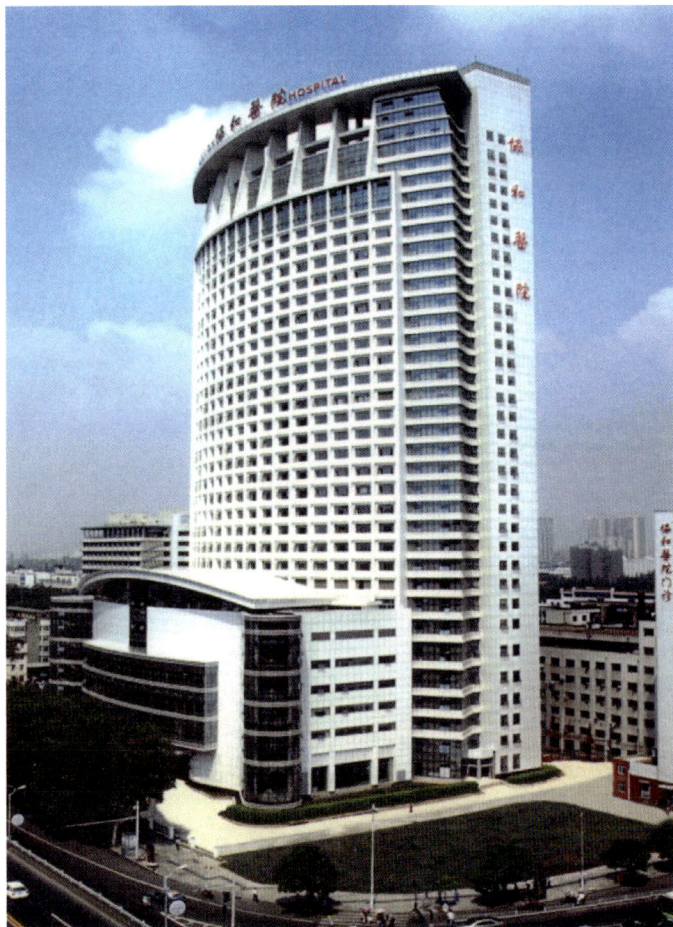

Figure 40

The new surgical block functioning today (Archives Wuhan Union Hospital 1866 – 2011)

I believe that, in spite of my historical account having so many imperfections, this record should be available to the large number of past and present employees at the Union Hospital. In October 2012 the author was privileged to present the substance of this history at an open meeting. By that time there were about 4000 employees of all walks of life working in that fine institution.

If the readers of this story about the first eighty four years of the Union Hospital have gained an idea of the sacrifice, dedication and sometimes the narrow escapes by those early pioneers, then this whole project is worthwhile. I am very much obliged to President Guobin Wang, who is also Professor of Surgery at the Union Hospital of Tongji Medical College, of Huazhong University of Science and Technology, for many reasons. He has on no fewer than three occasions, made me and surviving members of the Gillison family very welcome at the various celebrations of the hospital since 2001. It is a matter of much regret that the two previous generations of Gillisons and their colleagues did not live long enough to see the changes and the fine spirit of care and hard work for the patients of Wuhan today.

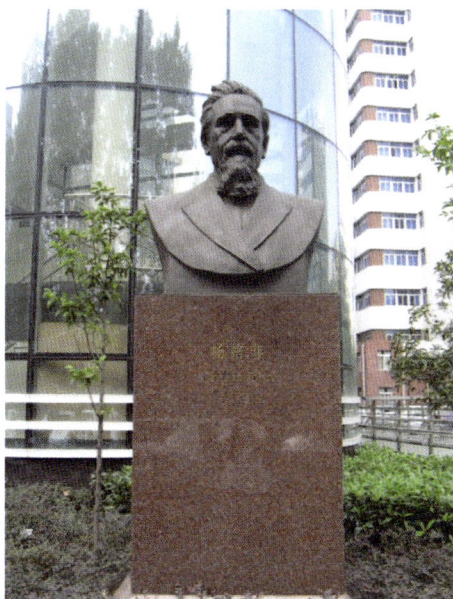

Figure 41
Griffith John's bust outside the
Modern Surgical block
(Photo by the author 2012)

It is symbolic that this fine bust of the founder Griffith John is placed in such a prominent position in front of the modern Union Hospital, thereby spanning 150 years. Griffith John would have been proud of all the events since 1866 and proud to see this thriving modern University hospital and Centre of Excellence today.

Walford Gillison

2015

REFERENCES

1. Thompson, R Wardlaw: Griffith John; The story of 50 years in China London The Religious Tract Society: Bouverie St & 65 St Paul's Churchyard EC (Popular revised edition 1908) page 162

2. Robson, William: Griffith John, Founder of the Hankou mission Central China; London SW Partridge & Co 8 & 9 Paternoster Row London page 87

3. Gillison, Keith: Personal communication to the author

4. Thompson R Wardlaw: Griffith John, The story of 50 years in China London The Religious Tract Society: Bouverie St & 65 St Paul's Churchyard, EC (Popular revised edition 1908) page 300

5. Ibid; page 205

6. Gillison, Keith: Personal reminiscence

7. Fluorens, PJ Hebd, C Seances Acad Sci Paris 1847; **24** 161, 253 and 340

8. Gillison, Keith: Personal communication (Anaesthesia in the tropics)

9. Jonathan D. Spence, "In Search of Modern China" pp 230–235

10. Clemmow, Frances: "Days of sorrow, Times of Joy. The story of a Victorian family's love affair with China" Metador 2012 page 180

11. Gillison, Keith "The Cross and the Dragon, a medical family in China"b Published and printed by Hawthornes of Nottingham 1988 page 21

12. Gillison, Kathleen: Personal communication through her 1929 diary

13. Clemmow, Frances: "Days of sorrow, Times of Joy. The story of a Victorian family's love affair with China" Metador 2012 page 234

14. McAll , Frances and Kenneth: "The Moon looks down" page 103

15. Report of the Union Hospital, Hankou 1929   Stored in the School of Oriental and African Studies (SOAS) London

16. Report of the Union Hospital, Hankou. 1930. Stored in the School of Oriental and African Studies (SOAS) London.

17. Gillison, Keith: "The Cross and the Dragon, a medical family in China" Published and printed by Hawthornes of Nottingham 1988 page 130

18. Report of the Union Hospital, Hankou 1932

19. Report of the Union Hospital, Hankou 1933

20. Report of the Union Hospital, Hankou 1934

21. Douglas, Beverley: Plastic and reconstructive Surgery 1936 **32:** Volume 5; pp 756 to 775

22. Report of the Union Hospital, Hankou 1935

23. Blanchard, C E: "The romance of proctology" Youngstown: Medical Success Press 1938: Chapter **6** 130-143

24. Gillison Keith: Personal communication

25. Report of the Union Hospital, Hankou 1936

26. Iris Chang: The Rape of Nanking (The forgotten holocaust of World War II) Penguin Books 1997

27. Auden, W H: Collected Shorter Poems 1930 -1944
London Faber & Faber 1950 ("In Times of War" XIX 279-280)

28. LMS, *Report of Union Hospital Hankow, 1937*, China Local Reports, CWML A3/3

29. Fenby, Jonathan: Chiang Kai Shek; China's Generalissimo and the Nation that he lost   Carroll & Graf Publishers, New York 2004 page 330

30. Chatterton, Jocelyn: "Protestant Medical Missionary Experience during the War in China 1937–1945: The Case of Hubei Province" PhD School of African and Oriental Studies, University of London Page 201 (*Nurses working all hours in city "Go Downs"*)

31. Ibid Page 190 (*Self help by refugees*)

32. Ibid Page 125 (*Changed relationships between Chinese and foreign workers*).

33. Ibid Page 203 (*Alleged "safety zones"*)

34. Letter of thanks to the Lord Mayor's appeal funds from the City of London (Archives of the School of Oriental and African Studies, London)

35. Orr, HW: Wounds and fractures: A clinical guide to Civil and Military Practice   Springfield Ill, Charles C Thomas 1941

36. Gillison, KH: An abduction splint used in war surgery in China Brit Med J 1940, 1 686-691

37. Chatterton, Jocelyn: "Protestant Medical Missionary Experience during the War in China 1937–1945: The Case of Hubei Province" PhD School of African and Oriental Studies, University of London page 219 (*Increased electricity cuts since Japanese occupation*)

38. Ibid page 221 (*Ingenuity of gypsum substitute from local sources*)

39. Report of the Union Hospital, Hankow 1940

40. Chatterton, Jocelyn: "Protestant Medical Missionary Experience during the War in China 1937–1945: The Case of Hubei Province" PhD School of African and Oriental Studies, University of London page 224-5 (*"Dr Chapman's providential "Hospital Stores Account"*)

41. Leck, Greg: "Captives of Empire: The Japanese Internment of Allied Civilians in China 1941-1945" Front cover

42. Chatterton, Jocelyn: "Protestant Medical Missionary Experience during the War in China 1937–1945: The Case of Hubei Province" PhD School of African and Oriental Studies, University of London page 244 (*Account of Dr J.K. Liu's accomplishments*)

43. Ibid page 354 (*The three principal reasons for Allied Internment*)

44. Chapman, HO: Report of the Union Hospital 1945

45. Harold Wickings in Rowlands, Edward "End of an era: Stories from Central China during the War Years" London Livingstone Press 1947

46. Chatterton, Jocelyn: "Protestant Medical Missionary Experience during the War in China 1937–1945: The Case of Hubei Province" PhD School of African and Oriental Studies, University of London pages 317-8 (*Antipathy of returning staff to those who remained*)

47. Gillison, Keith: "The Cross and the Dragon, a medical family in China" Published and printed by Hawthornes of Nottingham 1988 page 177

48. Gillison, Keith: personal communication to the author

49. Chatterton, Jocelyn: "Protestant Medical Missionary Experience during the War in China 1937–1945: The Case of Hubei Province" PhD School of African and Oriental Studies, University of London page 312 (*Urgent meeting of UNRRA, staff and ex-POW missionaries*)

50. Mao Tse Tung (1893-1976) 27/2/1957 Quotations of Chairman Mao 1966 page 302

ILLUSTRATIONS; OPIUM WARS.

APPENDIX 1

NOTES ON THE OPIUM WARS AND
CHRISTIAN MISSIONARY SOCIETIES

Introduction

I am not a professional historian but on the grounds of having been born in China, the son and grandson of missionaries to China, I have awarded myself the privilege of openly reading, thinking and commenting about the Wars and the implications for the various missionary societies. The first Opium war (1838 to 1842) took place between Britain and China, the second between Britain, France and the United States against China (1857 to 1860) which had far greater consequences.

The signing of the second war, the Tianjin (Tientsin) treaty in 1858, followed by the Beijing (Peking) treaty in 1860, hugely affected the whole missionary endeavour in China. People like the founder of the Wuhan Union Hospital, the Reverend Griffith John, had to wait in the Treaty port of Shanghai until he had the "Green Light" to venture into Central China to practise and convert people to his faith after that Treaty had been signed.

Both Jiang Jieshi (Chiang Kai Shek) and Mao Zedong (Mao Tse Tung) agreed that the years between 1839 and 1945 (including the second Sino-Japanese War) could be described as "One hundred years of Humiliation"[1]. Having studied the two wars I believe the evil of the Opium Wars should be recorded in all British history books today.

Once again the Pinyin terms will be used in this narrative. The Wade-Giles spelling will be put in parentheses on the first occasion, to be followed only by the modern Pinyin spellings afterwards.

PART ONE

OPIUM WARS SUMMARY

According to Fairbank[2], in the early part of the nineteenth century the Chinese foreign policy rested on three long-standing assumptions:

1. China's superiority in warfare

2. China's skill in "civilising" outsiders

3. The possession of precious trading goods to bring foreigners to accept the "tributary status"

Unlike China's Asian neighbours, the European powers refused to make these acknowledgements in order to trade. They demanded instead that China adhere to Western diplomatic practices including the creation of treaties. Although the "unequal treaties" and the use of the "most-favoured-nation" clauses were initially effective in creating and maintaining open trade with China, they were important factors in creating animosity and resentment toward Western imperialism[2]. Whatever happened to the negotiations in the middle of the nineteenth century the main players seldom got onto the same "wavelength" with each other.

While the Qing (Ching) Imperial dynasty believed that Chinese civilisation was superior to all others, so for a time exchanges of philosophy, religion and trade with other countries were not encouraged. For many years it was decreed that trade could only take place via the City and estuary of Guangzhou (Canton). As Chinese art, silk, porcelain, tea and other products stimulated increasing demand, it made western countries more eager to trade, but Chinese exporters usually required payments to be made in silver bullion rather than in the exchange of goods.

The opium poppy had been grown in China but addiction was not initially serious. In India cultivation of opium by the East India Company had become an expanding business in the nineteenth century for many years and for commercial reasons it really was serious. That particular Company was not permitted to trade directly with China until 1699. Officially the sale of opium for smoking was banned in China, but in India in 1829, where huge amounts of the poppy were grown, the seeds were stored and exported in increasing amounts.

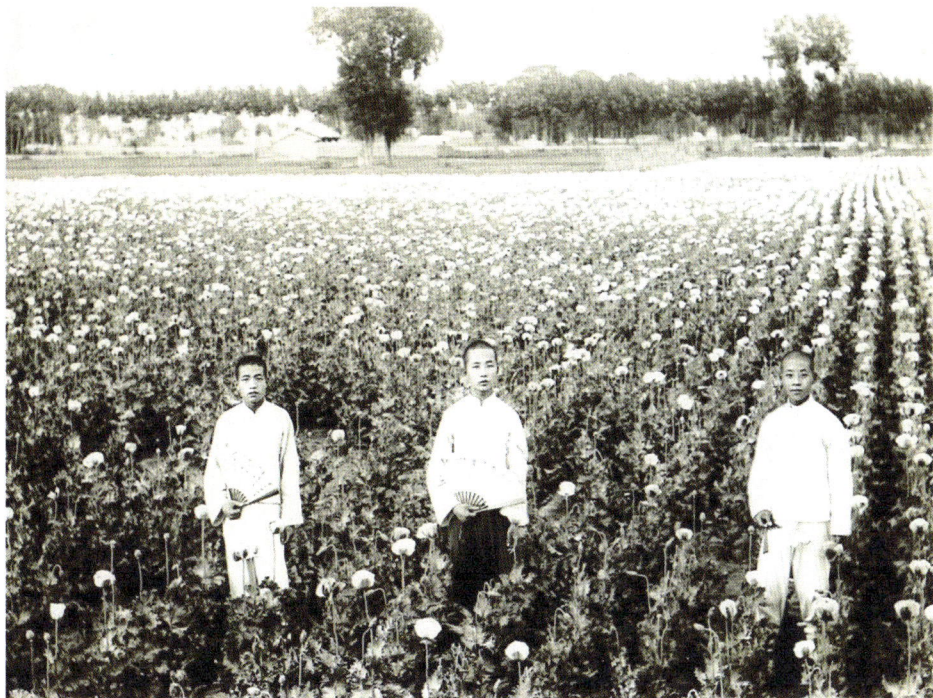

Figure 1

Contemporary opium poppy field and future victims
From "The Great Wen: A London blog 2013" Photo taken in 1899 used by an
Exhibition in London http://greatwen.com/category/drugs-2/

Figure 1 shows the picture of a typical crop of poppy plants growing
prolifically somewhere in China. Like the Chinese exporters, the East India
Company wanted to trade in silver bullion, but their contacts in London
preferred to exchange manufactured goods. Understandably during the
eighteenth and nineteenth centuries, while demand for tea and China
luxuries increased, Britain's silver resources steadily decreased.

From 1699 onwards, to offset the loss of silver, the East India Company
(supported by Britain) became involved in a lucrative trade of smuggling
opium from India into China. The prized Chinese exports were then
brought to Britain, the rest of Europe and the Americas (figure 2). The
mechanism of export into China was simple. Ships from the East India
Company would first bring the opium to storage ships anchored off-shore
from the Guangzhou mainland. Next, small fast boats run by local
entrepreneurs would collect and sell the banned material out of sight of the

authorities. Should any of those pirates be caught, the opium was burned, the vessel confiscated and very often the crew put to death.

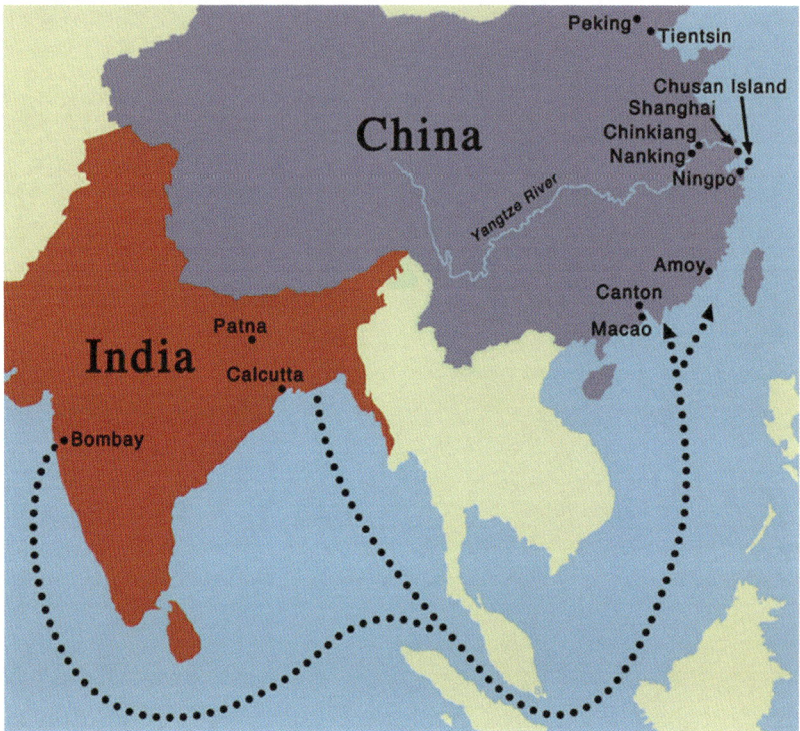

Figure 2

The lucrative trade routes of the East India Company about 1850
Peter C Perdue THE ANGLO-CHINESE WAR 1839-1842
Massachusetts Institute of Technology © 2010 Visualizing Cultures Creative
Commons License
http://ocw.mit.edu/ans7870/21f/21f.027/opium_wars_01/ow1_essay.pdf

Initially some sale of opium in China was permitted because opium in those days was then, as it is now, a valued medicine to relieve pain, assist sleep and, in limited circumstances, reduce stress. However the speed of opium imports leading to increasing levels of addiction for millions of Chinese raised alarms in the Qing government. The local militia was weak and ineffective against local rebellions due to opium addiction among the troops themselves. They turned out to be poor fighters. According to Spence,[3] if the believed figure of 10% of heavy opium smokers was correct, there would at that time be 15 million opium addicts in China (figure 3). To make matters worse trade officials became equally alarmed at the "rapidly increasing outflow of silver from China"[3].

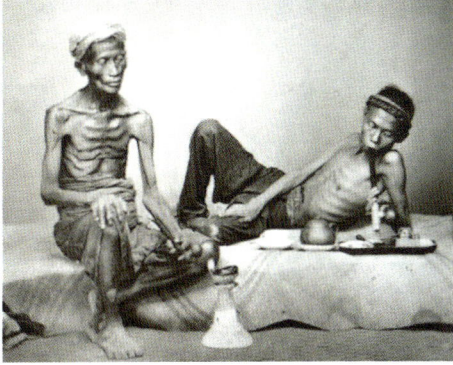

Figure 3

The sad sight of opium addicts with their pipes
From "Images for opium addiction in China"

It is no surprise the sales of opium were so lucrative that the East India Company ruthlessly continued to push further sales of opium into China (figure 4). As a result the very fabric of Chinese society was threatened.

Figure 4

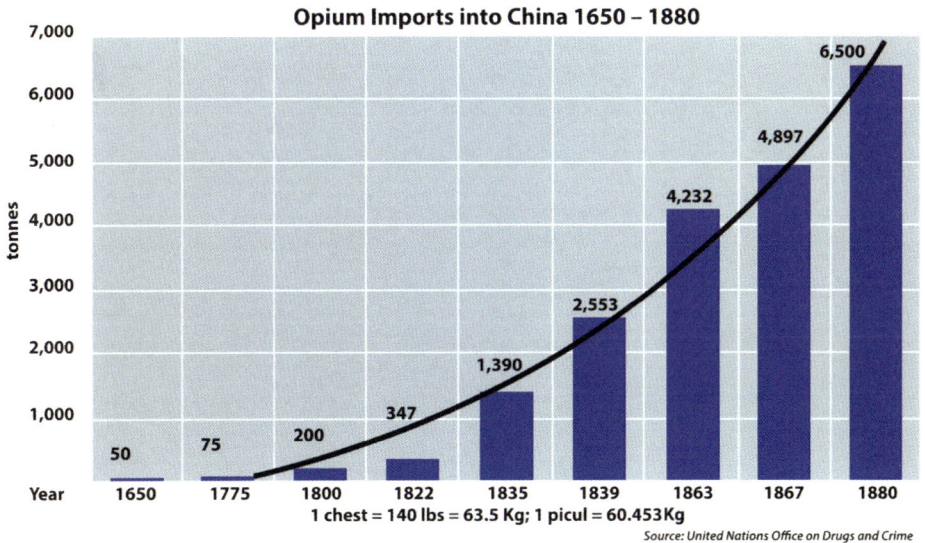

Opium Imports into China 1650 – 1880

1 chest = 140 lbs = 63.5 Kg; 1 picul = 60.453Kg

Source: United Nations Office on Drugs and Crime

en.wikipedia.org/wiki/History_of_opium_in_China

When the East India Company's trade monopoly was abolished in 1833, smuggling of opium into China by European private traders increased.

Much of the illicit trading took place around the Lintin Island which was just beyond the reach of jurisdiction of Guangzhou [4].

The First Opium War or "Anglo-Chinese War" 1838 – 1842

There were plenty of other grievances besides the "Opium boom" increasing the outflow of silver from China. It was obvious the 1838 Imperial decrees, supported by the Qing Emperor Daoguang, prohibiting the drug were being flouted. A new official of repute in the eyes of the Imperial Court was Lin Zexu[5] who was sent as a special commissioner to Guangzhou in March 1839. This new arrival was the son of a school teacher; he had a glittering career in the diplomatic service and was determined to deal with the crisis.

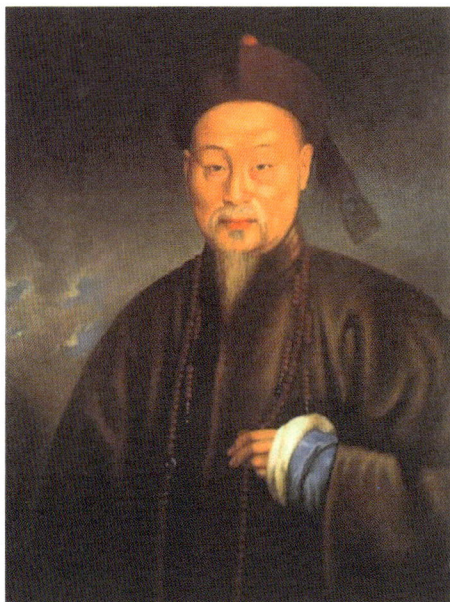

Figure 5

General Lin Zexu
Beinecke Library, Yale University
1800s_Lin Zexu_3454_001_Yale

On arrival in Guangzhou Lin took three major steps:

1. All smokers had to hand over their pipes
2. Besides banning illegal opium, he circulated his edict to the Chinese community and all foreigners including writing a pointed letter to the British Queen Victoria. There is no record the letter actually arrived at the Royal palace.
3. All foreigners' opium which was stored in Hongs (defined as foreign mercantile houses in China) was to be surrendered. Factories were closed and barred with 1000 guards installed while all streets to the

factories were closed. All the detained foreigners, including Captain Charles Elliott, the British Superintendent of Trade, were held hostage without food or personal servants for several days.

The deadlock was temporarily broken when Charles Elliott promised to purchase the confiscated 20 chests of opium worth £2 million at 1840 rates. This delighted the "Hongists" whose valuable stock had been frozen by General Lin. Elliott had to declare that the captives would swear to abandon the opium trade or risk capital punishment. He was also expected to promise to hand over a British seaman who had recently killed a man in Kowloon. This last promise he refused.

According to the British point of view these demands by General Lin were enough to precipitate the war against the Chinese authorities in Guangzhou. On the excuse of defending "Free Trade", Britain declared war against China in 1839 which continued until 1842. This war between China and Britain alone was known as the First Opium War.

The war turned out to be an unequal contest because of the superior fire power of the British Royal Navy and its marine forces. The new armoured steam ship "Nemesis" changed the whole pattern of the war because with its shallow draught it easily negotiated the channels of the Pearl River and its estuary. To his horror Lin Zexu confirmed that his army at many levels was addicted to opium; it was far from battle-ready thanks to easy access to the drug. Once the forces in Guangzhou had been isolated, and Hong Kong Island guarded, reinforced British troops were able to advance along the whole eastern coast of China also establishing bases at great speed along the Yangtse River and the Grand Canal. Fearing invasion at the seat of government in Beijing, the Qing government capitulated.

Imperial Commissioner Qiying, representing Emperor Daoguang, and British plenipotentiary Sir Henry Pottinger, acting on behalf of Queen Victoria, concluded their negotiations on August 29 1842 by jointly signing the Treaty of Nanjing (correctly described as an "unequal treaty") on board the British warship *HMS Cornwallis*.

Hence the Nanjing Treaty comprised some of the following factors:

1. Legalisation of the opium trade

2. Access to the five ports listed below, allowing unimpeded trade in their territory which were:

- Guangzhou
- Amoy
- Foochow
- Ningpo
- Shanghai

3. It allowed the inland tide of missionaries and other foreign groups to those ports and permitted them theoretically only a day's journey beyond the confines of each treaty port. In practice many missionaries flouted the edict and journeyed far further into China beyond the statuary day's journey.

4. It damaged the respect and fortunes of the Qing dynasty.

Added insult was inflicted by the "Supplementary Treaty of Bogue (Humen)" on October 8th 1843 which included:

- A huge monetary fine of 21 million silver dollars. The excuse was that the vanquished party had to pay for the costs of the war, including the three million dollars confiscated by General Lin in 1839.

- The permanent ceding of the island of Hong Kong to the United Kingdom. It was then a rocky island with a scattering of fishermen's huts on the shores of the island.

General Lin had been wrongly disgraced at the outcome of the war and dismissed. However his reputation was fully restored after his death; besides the corrections on the historic record, there is one fine statue of him in Guangzhou and another in New York.

In Britain the war was strongly criticised by the political party which was in opposition to the Government at the time. A young politician, William Gladstone, later to become Prime Minister, made the following statement in the House of Commons[6]:

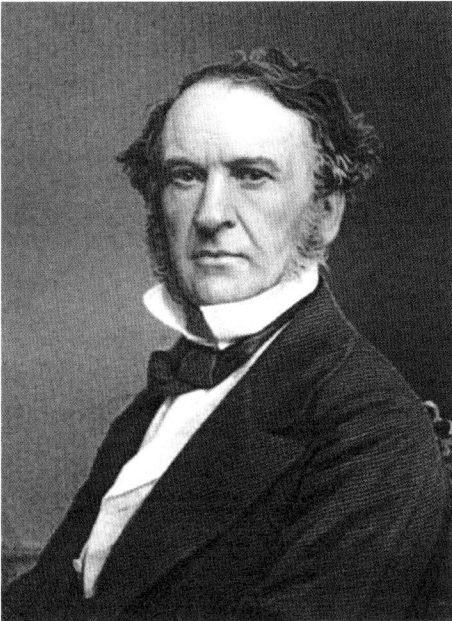

Figure 6

Portrait of William Gladstone

1809-1898
(Obtained from
"W.E. Gladstone images")

"How comes it to pass that the sight of the British flag always raises the spirits of Englishmen? It is because it has always been associated with the cause of justice, with opposition to oppression, with respect to national rights, with honourable commercial enterprise; but now the flag is hoisted to protect an infamous contraband traffic".

Other politicians, including Lord Palmerston, the Prime Minister at that time, claimed that opium was a relatively harmless habit and cynically said opium importation would help the balance of payments for both countries. Gladstone's Opposition colleagues managed to pass a vote of "no-confidence" in the government, precipitating a General Election but the patriotic fervour wrongly placed on the export of opium to China masquerading as "Free Trade" caused a landslide victory for Palmerston after the fresh election.

In the United States President John Quincey Adams[7] commented that opium was *"a mere incident to the dispute. . . the cause of the war is the kowtow, the arrogant and insupportable pretensions of China that she will hold commercial intercourse with the rest of mankind not upon terms of equal reciprocity, but upon the insulting and degrading forms of the relations between lord and vassal.".* Any President of the United States today would be horrified by such a comment.

To the more nobly motivated missionaries it meant at last they had access to other parts of China besides Guangzhou even though their access was gained on the back of such a military conflict.

Though not the first example, it was an example of "gun boat diplomacy" defined as "diplomacy conducted by threats of military intervention, especially by a major power against a then military weak state"[8]. This has been used in various ways by major powers ever since the 18th and 19th centuries; sometimes with subtlety, but mostly without.

The Second Opium War or "Arrow war" 1857 – 1860[9]

After quite a short while British merchants, aided by French and other national merchants, demanded more concessions than were granted by the Nanjing treaty. The final excuse to engage in a new war came in 1857 when some Chinese officials clambered on board the Steam Ship "Arrow" and lowered the British national flag. In fact the ship was a pirate Chinese ship sailing under a British flag of convenience. This event occurring within a short time after the murder of a French priest Auguste Chapdelaine in the interior of China gave France and Britain a further excuse for conflict.

It started with huge pressure from British and French naval shelling on the outskirts of Guangzhou, causing damage to civilian properties as well as fortifications. On the Guangzhou mainland and elsewhere many beheadings of foreigners took place. Conflict spread from Guangzhou and Hong Kong all the way up the coast, including Shanghai, right up to the Bay of Beihe close to Tianjin and Beijing (Peking). Heavy casualties by both armies were suffered near Tianjin; however the foreign troops had the advantage of new Enfield rifles which were quicker to load and had a more powerful range. The Qing government eventually surrendered as battles encroached nearer and nearer to Beijing.

At first Chinese Government representatives signed a second Tianjin treaty in 1858 shown in figure 7. Quite apart from this particular war, the Qing government was very much occupied with the infamous Taiping rebellion east of Shanghai, throughout a large part of lower Yangtse basin, and in the south all at the same time.

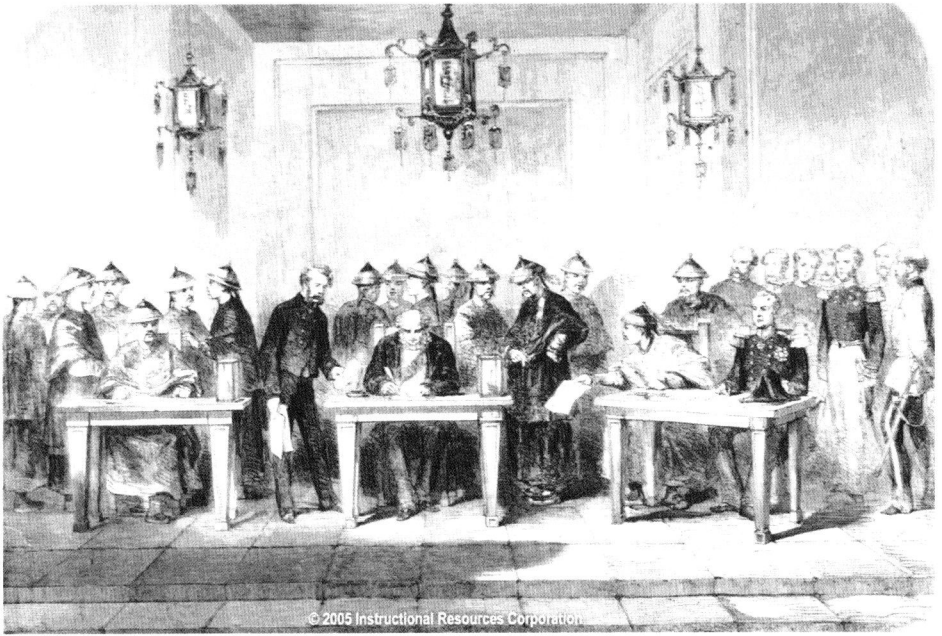

Figure 7

Signing of the Tientsin Treaty.
Getty Images. Universal Images Group.

The signatories were the British representative Sir Henry Pottinger and the Qing representatives, Qiying, Yilibu and Niujian. Emperor Xianfeng was furious about this, supported by a tough cabinet around him, so fighting continued after the signing for two more years.

Near to Beijing Lord Elgin sent 39 troops under a flag of truce to end the conflict. Regrettably these were captured and subjected to torture until liberated by French troops who found 18 dead and only 21 survivors. In retribution the British and French forces razed the beautiful Summer Palace with all its treasures to the ground, which has since been kept as a permanent monument to foreign desecration (figure 8).

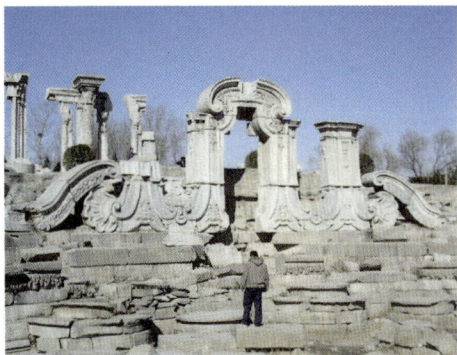

Figure 8

Remaining relics of the wrecked Old Summer Palace (Yuanming) garden
www.chinayak.com/Beijing/What-to-see-in-Beijing/Yuan-Ming-Yuan---Old-Summer-Palace.html

A decisive battle closer to the capital was won by Lord Elgin's forces with French help, so a more meaningful Treaty of Beijing followed in 1860. In the heat of the conflict around Beijing the Emperor Xianfeng fled the city, leaving his half-brother Prince Gong to ratify the Tianjin Treaty by signing the Convention of Beijing which really ended the war on October 18th 1860.

The foreign country to benefit the most was Imperial Russia who did not need to fire a shot. Thanks to threatening behaviour by the Russian envoy Ignatieff while British and French troops were still in Beijing, he got Prince Gong to sign a separate treaty conceding huge areas of land hundreds and thousands of square kilometres north of the Amur River corresponding to the size of Britain and France together and establishing the port of Vladivostok as a new port for Russia on the Pacific Ocean.

What were the results of this second Opium War? The major gains were:

1. Britain, France, Russia, and the United States would have the right to set up legations in Beijing, previously a closed city

2. Eleven more Chinese ports would be opened for foreign trade, including Newchiang, Tamsin (Taiwan), Hankou (Hankow), Tianjing and Nanjing. In the city of Tianjin itself there were no fewer than eight concession zones: Austro-Hungarian, Italian, Russian, Belgian, Japanese, German, British and French. The designation of concessions in Hankou is clearly shown in figure 9 below showing prize locations on the Yangtse River. The concessions are seen in the top right corner of the map.

   There was a difference between a "concession" and a "settlement". The term "settlement" refers to a parcel of land leased to a foreign power which is populated by both foreign and national peoples with locally elected foreigners governing them. The term "concession" refers to a long-term lease of land to a foreign power where the foreign nation has complete control of the land; it is governed by consular representation.

3. The right of foreign vessels including warships to navigate freely on the Yangtze River

4. The right of foreigners to travel into the internal regions of China for the purpose of travel, trade or missionary activities

5. China was to pay an indemnity to Britain and France in 2 million taels of silver respectively, and compensation to British merchants in 3 million taels of silver. In those days a British pound corresponded to three taels.

6. Official letters and other documents exchanged between China and Britain to be banned from referring to British Officials and Subjects of the Crown by the character (yí), meaning "barbarian"

Below is a map of Hankou, part of the greater City of Wuhan, which was one of the new city ports or territories granted by the Tianjin Treaty.

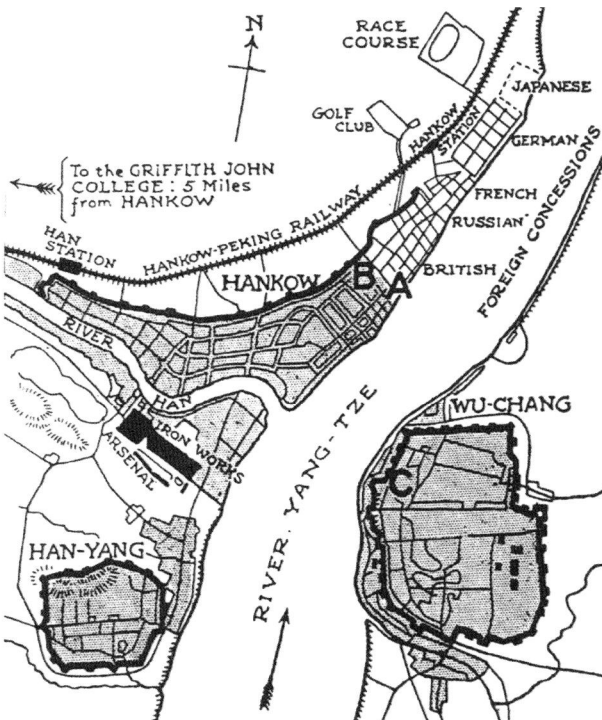

Figure 9

The three divisions of Wuhan as drawn in 1904

Thompson, R Wardlaw: Griffith John, The story of 50 years in China London The Religious Tract Society: Bouverie St & 65 St. Paul's Churchyard, EC (Popular revised edition 1908)

When the fighting was essentially over there appeared a Cartoon in a French journal showing the main players taking advantage of the predicament of the Government of China in 1860 in order to divide up the country between them (figure 10)."Chine" is the French word for "China".

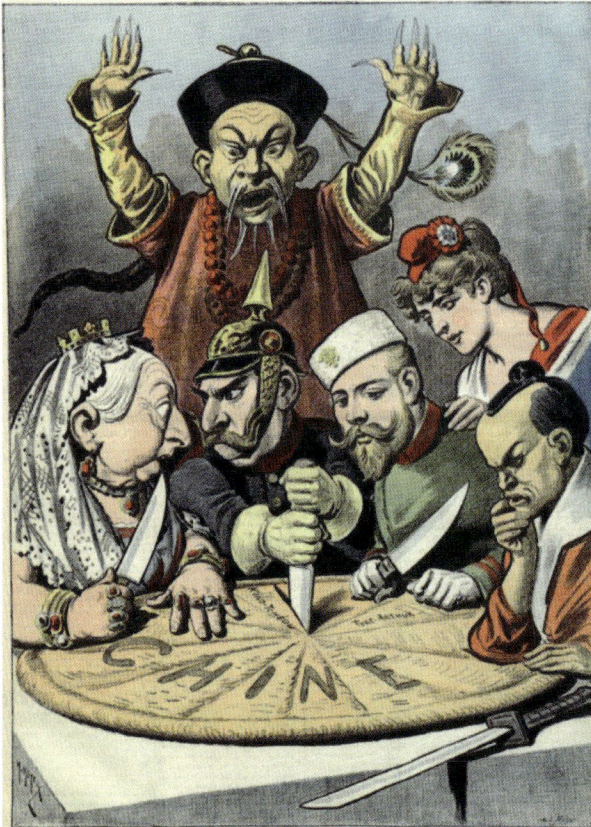

Figure 10

Cartoon devised by General Cousin-Montauban depicting the spoils of the Second Opium War Images from Second Opium War "Infiniti 2013" Designed by Studiopress. Sponsored by SSB Interview and wpspeak.com

(Left to right: Queen Victoria of Great Britain, Otto von Bismarck of Germany, Tsar Nicholas II of Russia, the Symbolic figure of France and Emperor Kōmei of Japan.)

What did the Missionary societies think about all this? Missionaries like Griffith John working in the Hankou, while glad to be able to travel freely around the country, were greatly saddened by the increasing number of opium addicts they encountered (figure 11).

1n 1858 he said in relation to Chinese resistance to the message of Christianity:

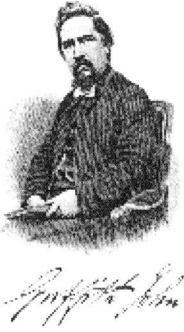

Figure 11
Griffith John 1831-1912

"The (opium) trade has damaged the Christian name in China to an extent hardly conceivable to people at home. Not only has it retarded the progress of Christianity by creating a strong prejudice against us; it has brought Christianity into contempt. As a people, the Chinese cannot distinguish between England and Christianity. Yet the acts of the British Government are supposed to be the expression of Christian morality."

A year later he continued: *"Opium smoking is the curse of China. The emaciated and ghastly appearance of these poor creatures is quite sickening* (figure 3). *It reaches all levels right up to the Emperor himself"*. The Reverend noted that the habit was less a cause of public shame since the early days of 1840. He and his colleagues were alarmed at the rapid spread of the addiction to which he said: *"Sadly the opium dens are now opened in broad daylight in every street; they are frequented from early morning to the late evening. The shame is now taken away by the universality of the practice. This is a fearfully black spot on our country"*. By that he implied that ordinary Chinese citizens understandably blamed the abominable spread of opium addiction on all foreigners especially the British[10].

PART TWO

MISSIONARY INVOLVEMENT BEFORE AND AFTER THE WARS

The first incursion was during the Tang dynasty in AD 635, when missionaries from the Church of the East (the Persian branch, cut off from the main church due to political tension between the Roman and Persian empires) came to China overland. This church was described as 'Nestorian' as it followed the doctrines of Bishop Nestorius, declared heretical in AD 431. Nestorianism flourished for a while in China but did not outlast the Tang dynasty owing to persecution in AD 845. Traces of Nestorianism have been seen in peripheral areas such as Mongolia.

The second time Christianity came to China was during the Yuan or Mongol dynasty (AD 1271-1368), when the Franciscans were commissioned by the

Pope in 1294 to carry out missionary activities in China. This second infusion of Christianity failed to survive the end of the Yuan dynasty.

The third wave came at the end of the Ming dynasty (AD 1368-1644), when a branch of the Roman Catholic Church known as Jesuits found their way to Beijing via Canton. The most famous of these was Matteo Ricci (1552-1610), an Italian mathematician who came to China in 1588 and settled in Beijing in 1600 (figure 12). Ricci was welcomed at the imperial court and also introduced Western learning into China. The Jesuits followed a remarkable and successful policy of accommodation to the traditional Chinese practice of ancestor worship, which was condemned by the Pope in Rome at the prompting of the Jesuits' enemies. Other Catholic missions failed to enjoy the same success.

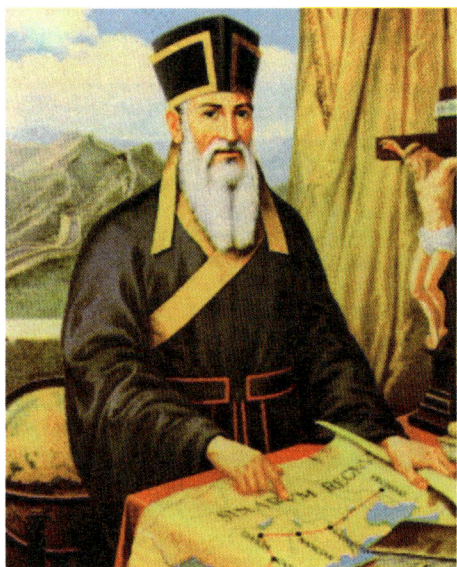

Figure 12

Matteo Ricci

Pages.uoregion.edu/inaasim/
qinglong/MingQing/Jesuits.htm

Further waves of missionaries came to China in the Qing (or Manchu) dynasty (1644-1911) as a result of contact with foreign powers. Russian Orthodoxy was introduced in 1715 and Protestant churches began entering China in 1807. What cannot be denied is that the First Opium War enabled a rapid increase of missionary incursion. Christian missionaries and their schools, under the protection of the Western powers, went on to play a major role in the Westernisation of China in the 19th and 20th centuries[12].

Merchants, soldiers and diplomats came to China to make a profit. Christian missionaries ostensibly came to give their services and on many occasions gave their lives for their beliefs. Robert Morrison (figure 13) arrived in 1807. Although he made few converts he compiled a Chinese-English dictionary and translated both the Old and New Testaments with the help of a colleague called William Milne. The spread of Christian religious literature followed in great numbers as a result of their efforts.

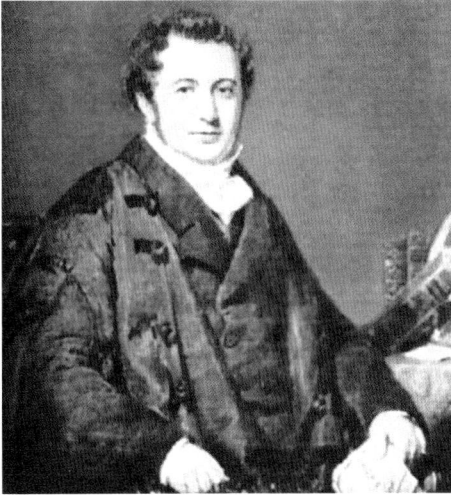

Figure 13

Robert Morrison (1782-1834)
First translator of the Old and New Testaments of the Christian Bible into Chinese
Newworldencyclopedia.org/entry/File: Robert_Morrison_1807.jpg

The founder of the China Inland Mission (CIM), James Hudson Taylor (figure 14), arrived in 1866 and immersed himself and colleagues in all things Chinese. Unlike the majority of missionaries, he and many CIM missionaries deliberately wore Chinese clothing in China.

Figure 14

James Hudson Taylor (1832-1905)
Founder of the
China Inland Mission
En.wikipedia.org/wiki/
Hudson_Taylor

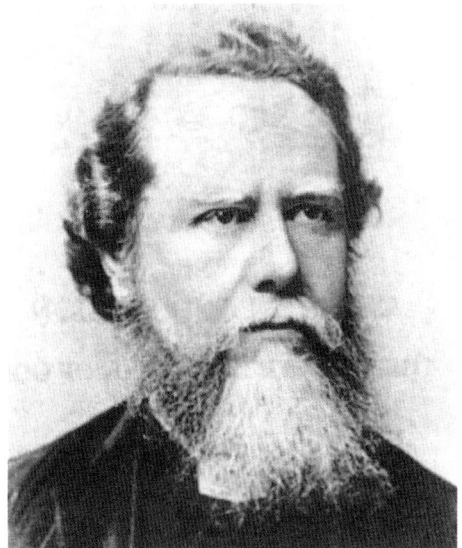

He understood the causes of the Boxer Rebellion, accepting that they were partly a reaction to the Opium Wars which he had publicly criticised both before and since. The CIM suffered badly during the Rebellion when 58 of their own missionaries, including 21 children, were killed.

In 1860 after the second Opium War there were 50 missionaries, including their children, living and working in China. Forty years later there were 2500 foreign missionaries, including 1400 British, 1000 American and 100 missionaries of Scandinavian origin. Needless to say, after the political changes from 1949 to 1950, there were no missionaries in China[5] after 1953.

Why were so many missionaries despised or even hated? On reflection it could well be because they wanted to change the culture of the people they encountered. Viewed by some it was psychologically iconoclastic. Perhaps the local Chinese suspected scorn poured on Confucianism and the harmless worship of ancestors. Later generations of missionaries like my parents had some respect for Confucianism and Taoism.

Western-style Medicine was a useful means of gaining influence in parts of China. There were only 10 western-style doctors in 1874 but 300 in 1905. A typical mission station would include[12]:

1. A preaching Hall or street chapel

2. Separate boys and girls schools

3. Secure residences for missionaries

4. Eventually a hospital such as the Union Hospital in Wuhan

Foreign hospitals escalated in 30 years but at least 300 Chinese doctors had been fully trained thanks partially to the number of textbook translations. Like it or not Christianity did gain more influence after the Second Opium War. Like Griffith John above, an overwhelming majority of missionaries and their Societies were horrified that the import of opium had enhanced their means of access to the whole of China. For example in 1891 opium addiction provided the highest cause of bed occupancy in the Union Hospital. Again in 1934 it was stated in a medical conference held in Nanjing that opium addiction was still one of the largest causes of bed occupancy in the state of Hubei. In Kathleen Gillison's 1934 diary she said there were no fewer than 56 opium dens in Hankou alone, quite apart from others in Wuchang and Hanyang.

As regards the Tianjin Treaty, it had to be admitted the Treaty gave all foreigners including missionaries the benefit of owning property, permission to travel and the ability to work in schools and hospitals. Without the Treaty they might have had to wait several decades. One misguided missionary, Michael C Lazich, said the Treaty might have been God's plan to allow entry of missionaries like himself into China[13]. The majority of missionaries such as Benjamin Broomhall, the president of the China Inland Mission who founded the "Anti-opium League in China", said in 1899: "The League provided the opportunity to state its abhorrence at having access into China on the back of the dirty Opium war"[14].

A public statement was made by 11 Missionary Societies, admittedly 85 years after the Tianjin Treaty. Quoted below are the two resolutions prepared by the Standing Committee of the conference of British Missionary Societies on October 6th 1925 and endorsed by the Baptist Missionary Society General Committee in November the same year. Its timing followed the Boxer Rebellion in 1900 and the residual anti-British and anti-Western feelings over the years. The Missionary Societies, led by the Baptist Missionary Society, felt that there was a huge need to apologise publicly for the unfair trade and military concessions squeezed out by European and American powers after the two Opium wars of the previous century.

1. *The under named British Missionary Societies working in China wish to make it known that they do not desire that the legal rights of their missions and missionaries in China should in future rest upon existing treaties between Great Britain and China. In particular upon the so-called toleration clauses in these treaties dealing specifically with missionary work, and they desire that their future rights and liberties be those freely accorded to them by China as a Sovereign Power and mutually agreed upon in equal conference between China and other nations.*

2. *The under named British missionary Societies note with satisfaction the announcement of His Majesty's Government of their readiness to join in steps towards a comprehensive revision of existing treaties between Great Britain and China. So far as the interests of missions and missionaries are concerned, they would welcome the abolition of the present articles relating*

to extra-territoriality and the substitution for them of such provisions for the administration of justice and the protection of the life and property of British nationals as may be mutually agreed upon in equal conference between China Great Britain and other powers.

The Societies approving these resolutions were:
1. The British and Foreign Bible Society
2. The China and Inland Mission (CIM)
3. The Society for the Propagation of the Gospel
4. The Church Missionary Society
5. The Wesleyan Methodists
6. The United Methodists
7. The London Missionary Society (LMS)
8. The Baptist Missionary Societies
9. The English Presbyterians
10. The Friends Foreign Missionary Association
11. The Zenana Missionary Society of the Church of England

These were noble sentiments but it is hard to judge how the sentiments affected the people of power in high places. The land settlements in the regions of all the old and new ports of admission lasted for many years almost up to the beginning of the Second Sino-Japanese War (1937–1945). Germany was deprived of its land concession in 1917, Russia relinquished its concessions in 1925, Britain in 1927 and the Japanese and French concessions remained until 1937. However Hong Kong remained a British Protectorate until the official handing over of the island and the New Territories in 1997.

An uninformed reader might well ask about the purpose and role that Christian missionaries of all denominations played in China. Why were they there? Missionaries have been out to China over 1500 years with varying lengths of stay. As described earlier, Christianity came to China not once but on several occasions.

The basic premise before was, and remains today, not only in the belief of God the Creator of the Universe, but also the belief in a personal God who has the power to influence each member of the human race. This God they believe can affect the lives of people they meet as well as provide a code of conduct for the society around them. The majority believed in an after-life called Heaven on dying; so important was this to them that they felt very strongly their purpose (hence the word "mission") was to convey this message to the whole population of China. Specifically some of these mostly well-intentioned people believed that their personal God wanted them to live and work in China for most if not all of their lives. Many died from infectious disease soon after arrival and some died from violent means such as after the Boxer Rebellion. Despite these life threatening hazards all of them believed that they were doing God's will.

It must be clearly said here that foreign governments did not pay any missionaries one single cent of their salaries for being out there. Having been the son and grandson of China missionaries I can confirm that to be true. The modest salaries of all the missionaries came from hundreds of varying sized donations; some were generous but many donations were very small, mostly from members of the home churches that had sent them out to China. The salary of a doctor was exactly the same as for a preacher, teacher or administrator when abroad. Many (not just members of the Medical profession) could have earned more if they stayed in their home countries.

At first the new Government of Chairman Mao, which had captured the whole of China apart from Taiwan in the 1949-1950 Civil war, permitted a gradual transfer of management of schools, universities and hospitals from European and American missionary hands to take place over a period of five years. The plan for a gradual transfer ceased abruptly at the outbreak of the Korean War on June 25th 1950[15]. All foreigners who were not members of the Communist Party had to leave China immediately. Missionaries Arthur Matthews (an American) and Dr Rupert Clark (British CIM) were placed under house arrest in Shanghai but were finally allowed to leave in 1953. Thus the China Inland Mission (CIM) was the last Protestant missionary society to leave China[15].

In 1900 there were an estimated 100,000 Chinese Protestant Christians in China. By 1950 the number had increased to 700,000, an impressive number but still far less than one percent of the total Chinese population. Helped by strong leaders such as John Sung, Wang Ming-Dao, and Andrew Gih, the Chinese Protestant Christian churches became an indigenous movement.

Summary

There is no doubt today that the Opium Wars were thoroughly evil and selfish acts enforced by the merchants and politicians of the day. Many missionaries like Griffith John (quoted above) were saddened and disgusted with the actions of the British Government.

The cost in human lives was heavy from time to time in the Mission field. Following the death of the French priest Auguste Chapdelaine in 1858 and others afterwards, it is estimated that about 250 missionaries were killed by the members and sympathisers of the Boxer Rebellion at the turn of the twentieth century. One must not forget that nearly 2000 Chinese Christians were killed at the same time. Why did such genocide take place at that time?

1. The confusion, stated by Griffith John, in the Chinese population in distinguishing well meaning, well motivated missionaries trying to help the local population from the greedy opium importers
2. Forty years since the signing of the Tianjin treaty is not a long time in adult people's lives; settling such a longstanding sore could well have encouraged revenge for the Opium Wars

There are accounts from all over China of bright, highly qualified and motivated young missionaries who died within a few days, weeks or months from infectious disease on arrival. Most if not all of them knew the risk to their lives from such a cause and that must have been considered by these pioneers. According to Jessie Lutz in the nineteenth century, as many as 50% of the missionaries died or resigned for reasons of ill health after 10 years of service and the infant mortality was three times higher than their contemporaries in the U.K.[16].

Not all the dangers came from infectious disease in more recent times. I clearly remember as a boarder in Britain the boy sleeping in the next bed to me in the dormitory lost his medical missionary father (Harry Wyatt) who was shot dead because he was mistakenly thought to be Japanese, in Tai-Chou in North China during the conflict between Chinese guerrillas and Japanese troops in 1938.

Yes, it is true missionaries got into China on the backs of the unscrupulous business tycoons and politicians following the Opium wars. Yet it must be said that because of their belief in a God of creation who was also their personal God, they felt compelled to live, work, play and if necessary die for their Chinese colleagues and compatriots in China. The evidence of schools, universities and hospitals founded by these missionaries provides a permanent record of some of the better by-products that followed the notorious Opium Wars.

Walford Gillison

2015

(Son and Grandson of missionaries to China 1882 - 1950)

References

1. Wang Zheng: "Never forget National Humiliation: Historical Memory in Chinese Politics and Foreign Relations" Columbia University Press ISBN: 978-0-231-14891-7

2. Fairbank, JK: The Cambridge History of China 10 page 174

3. Spence, J: Opium smoking in Ch'ing (Qing) China in "Conflict and Control in late Imperial China" 143 – 173 Editors Frederick Wakeman Jnr and Caroline Grant 1975

4. US Department of State: Office of the Historian

5. Bickers, R: "The Scramble for China; *Foreign Devils in the Qing Empire 1832-1914*" Penguin Books 2011 pages 75-78

6. (Quote by Gladstone) Holt, E: "The Opium Wars in China" Puttnam London 1964 pages 98-99

7. The Opium Wars still define relations between the UK and China. Pity the hapless Mr Cameron. By Julian Kossoff World Last updated: November 10th 2010 (Reference President Quincy Adams)

8. Collins English Dictionary - Complete & Unabridged 2012 Digital Edition William Collins Sons & Co Ltd 1979 1986 © HarperCollins Publishers 1998 etc

9. Cavendish, Richard: "History Today" Volume: 58 Issue 6 2008

10. Thompson R Wardlaw: Griffith John, The story of 50 years in China London The Religious Tract Society: Bouverie St & 65 St Paul's Churchyard, EC (Popular revised edition 1908)

11. Barbaric destruction or symbolic retribution – The Razing of the Yuanming Yuan Fondation Napoléon 2008 (article by Komlosy Anouska , former curator of Asian ethnography at the British Museum)

12. Cohen, Paul A: The Cambridge History of China 11 page 509

13. Lazich, Michael C: "American Missionaries and the Opium Trade in Nineteenth Century China" *Journal of World History* Vol. 17 No. 2 June 2007   pages 210-211

14. Lodwick, Kathleen L: *Crusaders against Opium: Protestant Missionaries in China, 1874–1917*, Lexington: University Press of Kentucky 1996

15. Gillison, Keith: "The Cross and the Dragon, a medical family in China" Published and printed by Hawthornes of Nottingham 1988 page 177

16. Lutz, Jessie G: "Attrition Among Protestant Missionaries in China, 1807-1890" *International Bulletin of Missionary Research* Vol 36 No. 1 January 2012 pages 22-27

ILLUSTRATIONS; Second Sino-Japanese War.

APPENDIX 2

THE SECOND SINO-JAPANESE WAR
Calendar of events

Once again the Pinyin terms will be used in this narrative. The Wade-Giles spelling will be put in parentheses on the first occasion, to be followed only by the modern Pinyin spellings afterwards.

FIRST SINO-JAPANESE WAR: Summary

The first Sino-Japanese War took place from August 1st 1894 until April 17th 1895. The peninsula of Korea had always been a bone of contention between China and Japan, ending up at the end of the 19th century with Korea being occupied by the joint-holding by both Chinese and Japanese military forces. In those more imperialistic times it was no surprise that one of those powers should want to have complete control of the Korean peninsula.

Over the previous millennium, invasions by Japan had taken place from Korea and likewise Korea had been used as a launch pad for conflicts by China against Japan. In 1894 there were far more Chinese soldiers on the ground, but Japan's forces were better trained in modern military technology. Added to that most of the battles were sea battles favouring the better equipped Japanese Navy. The war ended when the invading Japanese troops got closer and closer to Beijing (Peking) prompting the capitulation by the Qing leaders. The Chinese losses were about 35,000 troops from death or injury. The Japanese losses were about 5000[1]. In several accounts the death rate was higher from infectious disease than firepower.

SECOND SINO-JAPANESE WAR   1931 – 1945

Author's comment No writer in his or her right mind can possibly write a completely balanced summary of this vicious war. This summary is aimed at people concerned with the fate of Wuhan in Central China. Needless to say events that occurred hundreds or even a thousand miles away did affect the ordinary people of that city.

September 18th 1931 The Japanese manufactured an incident in Manchuria (originally part of North China) claiming the Chinese Army sabotaged the Japanese inspired and partly built South Manchurian Railway. Within 6 months a separate state from China called Manchukuo was proclaimed.

January 18th 1932 Five Japanese monks were attacked by a mob hired by the Chinese authorities resulting in the death of two monks in Hongkew, part of Shanghai. In addition a Japanese factory was burned to the ground. This provoked a Japanese retaliation by both land and sea from Japanese ships in the harbour, which did huge damage to the Chapei area of Shanghai.

January 28th 1932 A pitched battle between a Japanese naval landing party and the Chinese 19th Route Army took place.

February 27th 1932 The State of Manchukuo was announced by Japanese propaganda authorities. The deposed puppet Emperor Pu Yi was installed but the power remained very much with the military.

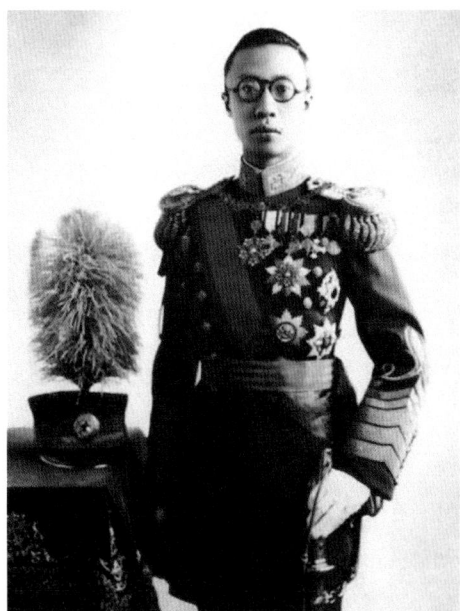

Figure 1

Emperor Pu Yi of Manchukuo 1931
(en.wikipedia.org/wiki/Puyi)

1933 Japan withdrew from the League of Nations.

November 25th 1936 The Anti-Comintern pact was signed between Japan and Nazi Germany against the "Third Communist International" movement that had been initiated by Stalin. The stimulus for the "Communist

International" was provided by Stalin who publicly supported China to reduce chances of Japanese invasion of the Soviet Union.

December 26th 1936 Jiang Jieshi (Chiang Kai Shek's) Kuomintang (KMT) party allied itself to Mao's China Communist Party (CCP) to resist the Japanese invasion.

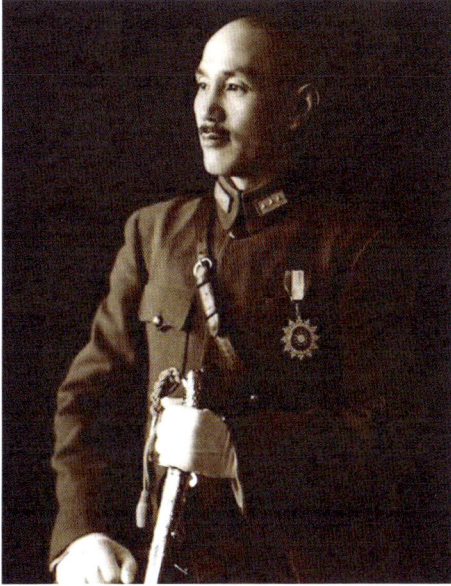

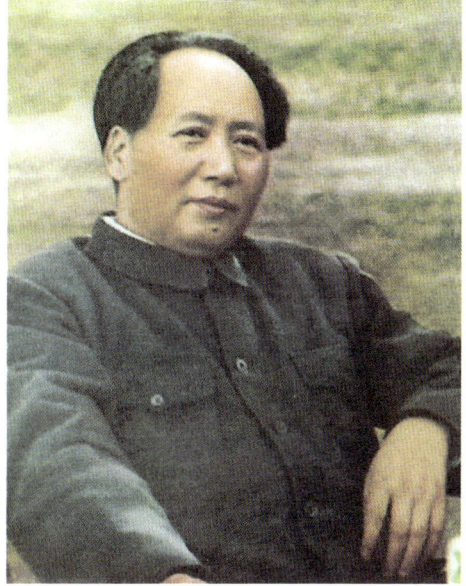

Figure 2

| **Jiang Jieshi (Chiang Kai Shek)** | **Mao Zedong (Mao Tse Tung)** |
| (Historyplanet.wordpress.com) | upload.wikimedia.org/wikipedia/ commons/0/0b/ Mao_Zedong_sitting.jpg |

July 27th 1937 A trumped up skirmish took place 10 miles from the outskirts of Beijing which was called the "Marco Polo Incident". Explanations varied from the disappearance of a Japanese officer allegedly due to assassination or absence simply because of his going to a toilet. Whatever the explanation the incident triggered the prompt invasion of the North Eastern Seaboard of China. The fall of Beijing and Tianjin (Tientsin) rapidly followed.

August 8th 1937 Aerial dogfights were evident for all to see taking place mainly over Shanghai.

August 12th 1937 A Japanese Naval officer was shot dead. This prompted the full invasion of Shanghai. Skirmishes took place all over the City. At least four suburban districts were badly destroyed by the combination of Japanese naval bombing and local Chinese army fighting. Many of Jiang Jieshi's crack troops fought a very determined battle causing many Japanese as well as Chinese civilian and military casualties. Shanghai eventually came under Japanese control after three months.

September 1st 1937 Stalin gives credits and loans to China. This was referred to as the "Sino-Soviet Non-aggression Pact".

December 13th 1937 This was the official date of the Fall of Nanjing, which had previously been a makeshift capital and military base for Generalissimo Jiang Jieshi. When Jiang realised he did not then have the land-army and air power to successfully resist the invasion he left for Wuhan further west. In Nanjing the official Commander of the Japanese forces (General Iwani Matsui) became ill for several days, so his next-in-command (Prince Asake Yasuhiko, an uncle of the Japanese Emperor) took over. This commander and troops were responsible for the rape and killing of hundreds of women with additional slaughter of up to 300,000 Chinese soldiers and citizens in seven weeks[2].

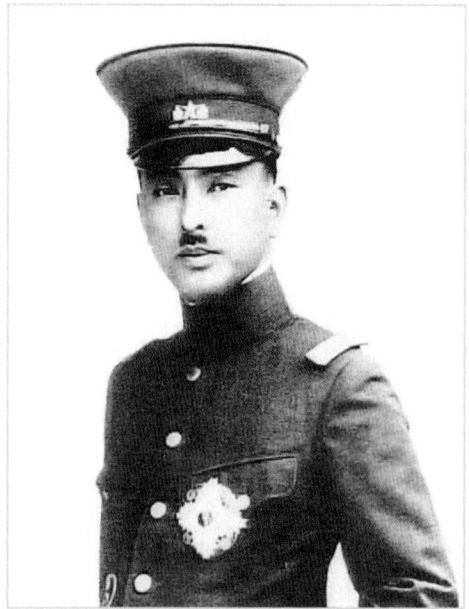

Figure 3

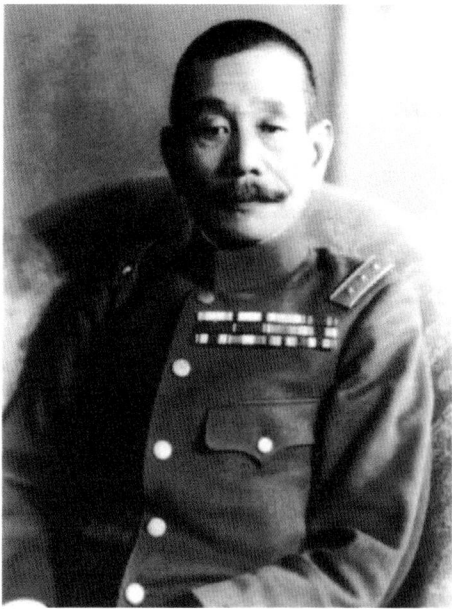

General Iwani Matsui   **Prince Asake Yasukiho.**
(Images from Wikipedia)

It was claimed at the War Crimes Commission that after he had recovered from his illness, General Matsui had written back to Japan to say how shocked he was with the news and that he deplored the carnage. He further claimed that when he reprimanded his immediate juniors, including Prince Asake, he was greeted with no contrition, merely laughter[3].

Further details are described[4] elsewhere of decapitation contests, bayoneting practice, thousands of rapes usually followed by killing, castrations, disembowelment and live burials. (Though many officers were taken to the War Tribunal courts in Japan after the war, General MacArthur had given the Royal Family an amnesty which included Prince Yasuhiko).

There were not one but two crimes in Nanjing:

> 1. The capture, rapes and slaughter
> 2. The cover-up afterwards

January 1st 1938 "Advent of the China Foreign Assistance Programme." This took place between the Soviet Union, United States, United Kingdom and France who between them gave $263 million US dollars aid to China.

Meanwhile throughout the following 6 months a three-sided war of attrition took place among the main contestants. On one side there was the Japanese Emperor, or more likely his war military cabinet, in the eastern part of China fighting to invade, and capture more and more territory further west. It was then mainly a guerrilla war against Mao Zedong (Mao Tse Tung) in the northwest and Jiang Jieshi in the South and West. It was not long before personal animosity and even military conflicts between Mao and Jiang took place in the last two years of the World War. Both Mao and Jiang knew a conflict would take place against each other when the war with Japan was over.

Added to the main contestants above there were smaller groups with their own agenda. There was a group of bandits who called themselves "The Loyal Patriotic Army" and a group near Shanghai called "The Pootung Pirates Association", both groups later proving they were well suited for underground activity throughout the war. In addition there was a "Quisling-style" group under ex-President Wang Qing Wei who hated Mao's CCP sufficiently to link up with Japan for most of the war.

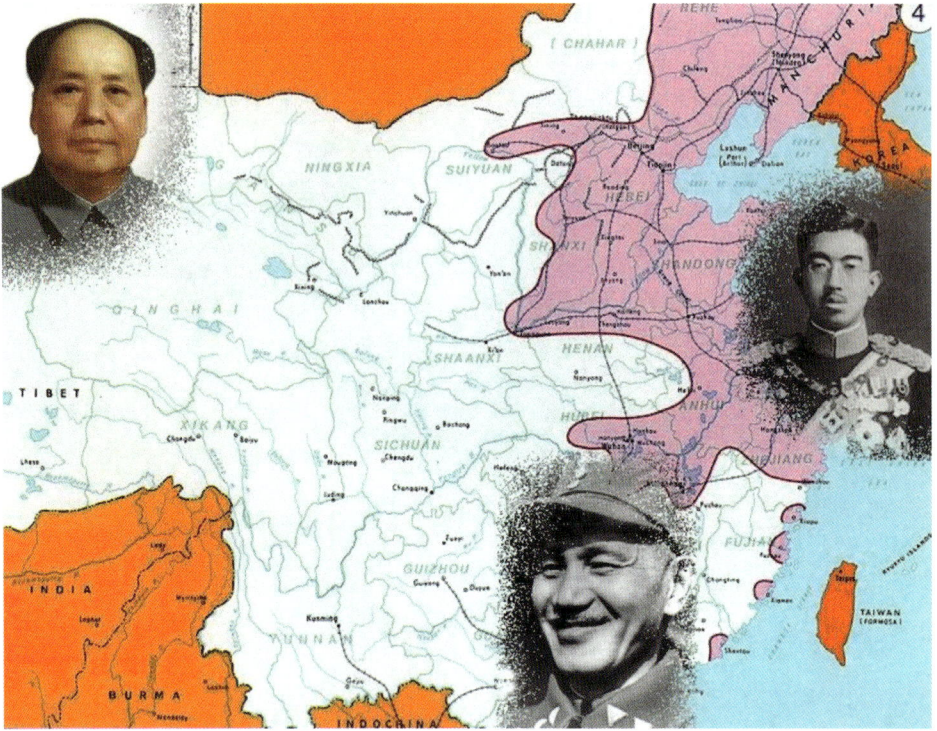

Figure 4
Main protagonists Second Sino-Japanese War
Author's own photo collection: note Taiwan was then Japanese territory

October 11th 1938   The beginning took place further east near Jiujiang (Kiukiang) with a fierce battle decided at the River Yangtse borders. Further fierce fighting occurred from high mountains nearby at Lushan (Kuling) which the Japanese bypassed after no initial success in the mountains.

August 19th to October 27th 1938 THE BATTLE OF WUHAN

The Japanese forces invaded the province of Hubei and steadily advanced further west towards Wuhan mainly along the Yangtse River aided by good naval military support. Meanwhile considerable bombing of Wuhan took place where Jiang had set up a provisional government.

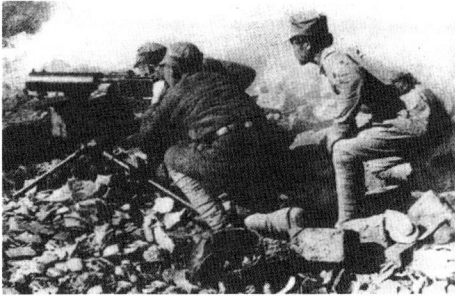

Figure 5

Chinese machine-gunners during Battle of Wuhan October 1938
en.wikipedia.org/wiki/Battle_of_Wuha
n#mediaviewer/
File:Wuhan_1938.jpg

Figure 6

Japanese troops entering Wuhan suburbs on October 17th 1938
ww2db.com/image.php?image_id
=18405

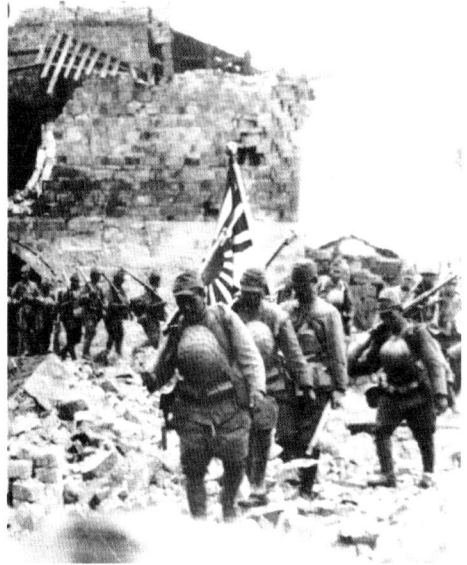

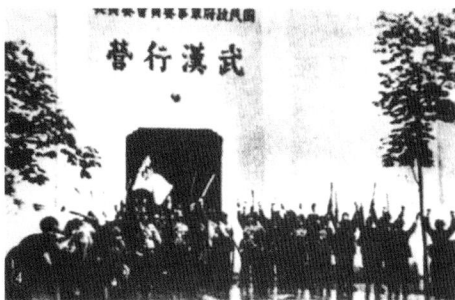

Figure 7

Japanese Troops celebrating capture of Wuhan military barracks October 27th 1938
wwiirazer.blogspot.co.uk/
2014/03/Battle-of-Wuhan.html
(Images from World War II database)

October 26th and 27th 1938 After many weeks of bombing, the time was ripe for the occupation of all of Wuhan by Japanese troops. Only a few days before, Jiang Jieshi's Kuomintang (KMT) and his Nationalist government had rapidly moved to Chongqing (Chunking) [4]. Japanese troops took over the whole city of Wuhan except for the foreign settlements. The puppet governor called Wang Qing Wei was appointed. His militia achieved greater significance at the end of the war.

Although the Japanese military claimed the battle a success because of its occupation of Wuhan, the cost of casualties for the Japanese was 140,000. Regrettably the cost in civilian and army lives in the Chinese population reached 400,000. Nevertheless the Japanese Government in Tokyo was frustrated by the consequences of the Battle of Wuhan because troops were not available to assist Japan in the Pacific war with America and Britain[5]. Not only that but in the last months of the war, there were no available troops to return to defend Japan, the Fatherland.

August 23rd 1939 Japan renounced the Anti-Comintern Pact because it was outraged by the new German-Soviet Union "Non-aggression Pact".

September 27th 1940 Japan acceded to the "Tripartite Pact" between Japan, Germany and Italy which implied mutual support among the three countries.

January 1st 1941 The New Fourth Army incident took place between the KMT and the Mao's China Communist Party (CCP) in a short skirmish. Until that time hostilities between Jiang and Mao had been suspended while they were officially united against the Japanese. That date signalled the end of real co-operation between the Nationalists and Communists.

June 1st 1941 Operation Barbarossa; Germany invaded USSR which distracted Soviet support for China.

December 7th 1941 The attack on Pearl Harbor took place. Japan was now at war with the United States.

December 18th 1941 Invasion and capture of Hong Kong followed. Japan was now at war with Britain, the British Empire and Commonwealth.

March 1st 1942 The China National Airlift Corporation was established. This enabled the beginning of supplies from India to China, mostly from "Burma Road" eastwards. Hundreds of flights were at risk from Japanese interception and dangerous weather conditions over the Himalayas, costing lives and aircraft delivering civil and military supplies to Jiang based in Chonqing.

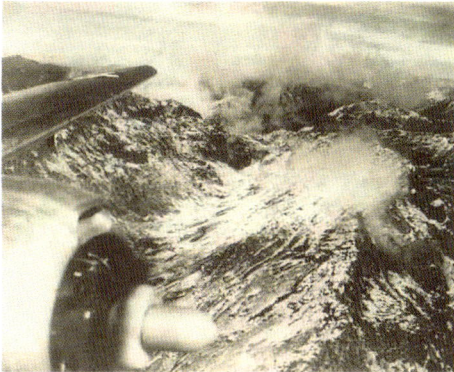

Figure 8

View over the Himalayas during flight of the Chinese National Airlift Corporation
Photo from Audrene and
Bob Sherwood
(U.S. Air force Photo)

February 15th 1942 Fall of Singapore. The British forces completely underestimated the speed, ferocity and hardened fighting ability of the Japanese who unexpectedly advanced from the peninsula of Malaya. The majority of defences were directed out to sea expecting a naval attack. They were not expecting an attack from the north of Singapore along a narrow difficult terrain.

November 1st 1943 The Cairo Conference. Churchill, Roosevelt and Jiang meet for the first time raising Jiang's status.

1944 – 1945 Renewed bombing of Wuhan, this time by Sino-U.S. aircraft, took place, signalling the reverse in the tide of war with Japan. Unfortunately the very busy though makeshift Ho Chi hospital in the middle of Hankou was bombed with some loss of patient and staff lives.

August 6th 1945 The first atom bomb dropped on Hiroshima. This disappointed Jiang who wanted the Allies to invade Japan conventionally from the China coast.

August 9th 1945 The USSR invaded and defeated Japanese troops in Manchuria. A second atom bomb dropped on Nagasaki.

August 14th 1945 Japan officially surrendered to the Allies on USS Missouri.

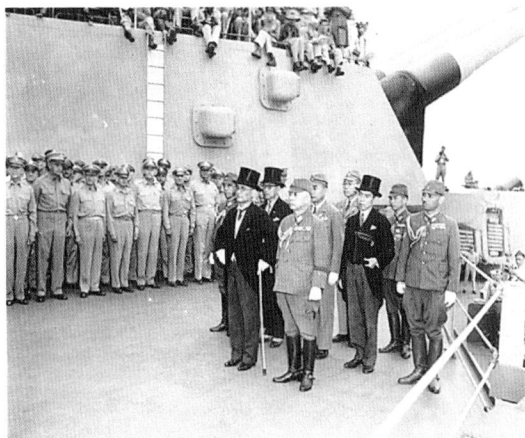

Figure 9

Japanese surrender signatories arrive aboard the USS Missouri in Tokyo Bay for the ceremony September 2nd 1945
www.google.co.uk/
search?q=Japanese+surrender+U
SS+Missouri&rlz

September 9th 1945

The formal Japanese surrender in the China Theatre took place only a week later in a simple 20 minute ceremony in the auditorium of the Central Military Academy in Nanking at 9.00 am on 9 September 1945. General Ho Ying-chen, Commander-in-Chief of the Chinese Army, received the surrender from Saburo Kobayashi who represented Lieut Gen Okamura Yasutsuji, Commander of the Japanese Forces in Central China, all representing their respective governments. Immediately following the signing of the Act of Surrender, General Ho handed Order No. 1 of Generalissimo Jiang to Lieut. Gen. Okamura as a supplement to the Act of Surrender.

Figure 10

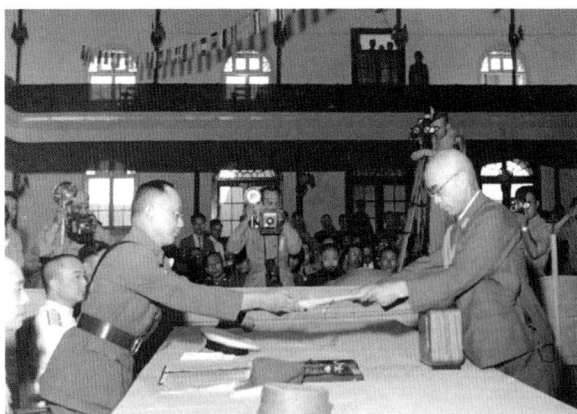

General Ho Ying-Chen He Yingqin , Commander-in-Chief of the Chinese Army (left) and Saburo Kobayashi, the representative of Yasuji Okamura the head of Japanese forces in China, handing over the surrender documents

gardnerworld.com/cbi/lens.htm

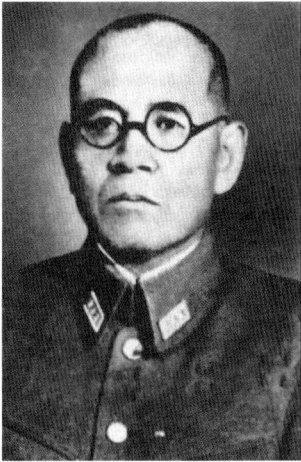

Figure 11

General Yasuji Okamura (Okamura Yasuji).
Supreme Head of the Japanese forces in China.

The reason for the non-appearance of General Yasuji Okamura is obscure for such an important occasion. Certainly there was a request from President Jiang to the Japanese General for him to stay in China and advise Jiang in the forthcoming Civil War that was inevitably coming between him and the CCP.

The USSR dismantled and imported most of the factories in Manchuria. The majority of Japanese weapons, mostly in the north of China, were surrendered to CCP Red Army.

Since 1931, what started as a series of serious skirmishes between those two countries along the eastern coast of China led to all-out war in 1937 when a large area of eastern and northern China, including the city of Shanghai, and the areas of that city beyond the limits of the International Settlement and French Concession, came under the control of the Japanese. After Pearl Harbor, Japan became involved in fighting the Allies on more than one front. This extended war was not only against its old enemy China, but against the Americans in the Pacific, the British in their Colonies and other countries in the Far East as they advanced into Burma towards India.

Contemporary studies from the Beijing Central Compilation and Translation Press have revealed that during the second Sino-Japanese War Japan suffered a total of 2,227,200 casualties, including 1,055,000 dead and 1,172,341 injured. These numbers were largely based on Japanese statistics[6].

References

1. Asianhistory.about.com/od/warsinasia/a/First-Sino-Japanese-War.htm

2. Chang, Iris: The Rape of Nanking (The forgotten holocaust of World War II) Penguin Books1997

3. Brackman, Arnold C: "The other Nuremburg" (William Morrow and Co Inc) pages 182 – 184 New York 1987

4. Fenby, Jonathan: Chiang Kai Shek; China's Generalissimo and the Nation that he lost.
Carroll & Graf Publishers, New York 2000 page 330.

5. Chen, C Peter: The Battle of Wuhan: Internet; World War II Database

6. Liu Feng, (2007).
Central Compilation and Translation Press
ISBN 978-7-80109-030-0
Note: This Chinese publication analysed the statistics provided by Japanese publications

APPENDIX 3

TEAMWORK FOR HEALTH IN CENTRAL CHINA. 1947

The proposed Central China Christian Medical Union. (CCCMU).

Summarised paper submitted by Keith Gillison FRCS Ed. and Hugh Owen Chapman M.B., B.T.M. This paper was a serious attempt for the complete co-operation between all medical centres to put away any private competition for revenue, but instead put up a very strong case for establishing a University Medical Centre

The report is prepared from the collaboration between:

1. The Union Hospital.
2. The Institute of Hospital Technology (I.H.T.).
3. The United School of Midwifery and Child Welfare.

BACKGROUND

Wuhan at the time of writing had a population of 1.5 million, situated 700 miles from the estuary of the Yangtse River and at high tide the river is about one mile wide.

It was prophesied that one day there would be a Hydro-electric plant near Ichang (Yichang). Thereafter there should be:

1. Cheaper electricity.
2. Better flood control.
3. Increased manufacture of chemical fertilisers.

MEDICAL ESTABLISHMENT

At the present time there is no university hospital, so the more specialised problems have to be referred to larger cities. Therefore there is a need for more medical training in all specialties.

At the time of writing in Wuhan there were:

Government beds..	360.
Military beds..	400.
Community Beds..	210.
Mission Hospital beds..	850.
Protestant Religion. 510.	
Catholic Religion. 340.	

The surrounding hospitals in distance vary from 40 to 180 miles away from Wuhan with even fewer beds between them.

Besides the Union Hospital in Wuhan were:

Church General Hospital. (China Inland Mission).
Methodist General Hospital.

With approaches already made to:

The Protestant Episcopal Church of America.
The Swedish Mission. (*Expertise in Radiotherapy in place*).
The United Church of Canada. (*Under Dr Robert McClure war-time expert in Flying Squad Medicine*).

To all these hospitals more trained doctors and nurses are expected.

The authors agreed there is a need to increase the number and the quality of the medical service. With so many beds, so many patients, midwives and technicians together; these would make an outstanding teaching centre worthy of university recognition.

The Union Hospital was founded in 1866 five years after Griffith John (London Missionary Society) arrived in Hankou. Dr Porter Smith started the Methodist General Hospital and Jubilee Hospitals in 1864 to be staffed by Methodist missionaries gradually handing over to Chinese doctors. Collaboration was agreed in 1925 and the building built in 1928.

The I.H.T. was also founded in 1928. From the start it trained technicians from all over China.

Plans have already been made for:

1. A new Head Physician for the Department of Medicine.
2. Head of Obstetrics and Gynaecology.
3. An overall Business Manager.

ASPIRATIONS

1. University recognition.
2. Operating theatres, X-Ray facilities, laboratories, private and general wards so as to admit all social strata.
3. While there are 200 to 250 beds for teaching available now, more are planned for the future.
4. A Medical Superintendent with Professorial chairs in Medicine, Surgery, Obstetrics and Gynaecology and Paediatrics. Appropriate junior staff levels are planned.
5. A Board of Management of Churches and businesses in the city.
6. Heads appointed for ability and unrelated to nationality.
7. All doctors to assist in teaching all trainees.
8. Proper medical records and medical library.
9. Regular medical meetings at all major sites in Wuhan.
10. All institutions to be based on Christian principles as priests or ministers have a role in patient recovery

....

THE INSTITUTE OF HOSPITAL TECHNOLOGY (I.H.T.).

As graduates have gone nation-wider after training, hostels are needed to house new trainees.
More staff needed to teach laboratory techniques.

....

MIDWIFERY

The school is already established in Wuchang.
It is a small start for a tremendous need.

At present there is only one British and one New Zealand obstetric teaching nurse staff so far.

....

CHINA'S NEED

Currently there are 15000 doctors in China which is 1: 30,000 patients. The patient: doctor ratio is about four times the ratio in the U.K.

Already Government Health Administration has made repeated requests to Mission Societies to help in training more Chinese doctors. (*Here the authors have made a strong plea for a spiritual emphasis*).

....

DRAFT CONSTITUTION

For the new University teaching hospital committee each hospital should provide:

- One Superintendent and one other.
- One representative of the School of Nursing.
- One representative of the I.H.T.
- One representative of the School of Midwifery.
- One representative from an outlying hospital beyond Wuhan.
- One representative of the Synod of Churches.
- One representative of the Business community.

Such a committee should:

1. Co-ordinate purchases of resources.
2. Be prepared to make recommendations on all matters.
3. Initiate appeals for help to any members.
4. Elect executive officers when necessary.
5. Alter the constitution democratically where necessary.

Keith H. Gillison.   *Henry O. Chapman.*

1947

INDEX